Shoulder Surgery - Open vs Arthroscopic Techniques

Edited by Dimitrios D. Nikolopoulos and George K. Safos

Published in London, United Kingdom

Shoulder Surgery - Open vs Arthroscopic Techniques
http://dx.doi.org/10.5772/intechopen.1000399
Edited by Dimitrios D. Nikolopoulos and George K. Safos

Contributors
Adrián Aziz Cortés de la Fuente, Maximiliano Cruz Palacios, Svetoslav Dobrilov, Raquel Guitián-Montes, Samer Amhaz-Escanlar, Alberto Jorge-Mora, Ana Carolina Presas-Presas, Matilde Delvecchio, Gian Mario Micheloni, Andrea Giorgini, Giuseppe Porcellini, Allyson Cabral, Paulo Veiga

First published in London, United Kingdom, 2023 by IntechOpen
IntechOpen is the global imprint of INTECHOPEN LIMITED, registered in England and Wales, registration number: 11086078, 5 Princes Gate Court, London, SW7 2QJ, United Kingdom

British Library Cataloguing-in-Publication Data
A catalogue record for this book is available from the British Library

Additional hard and PDF copies can be obtained from orders@intechopen.com

Shoulder Surgery - Open vs Arthroscopic Techniques
Edited by Dimitrios D. Nikolopoulos and George K. Safos
p. cm.
Print ISBN 978-1-83769-673-4
Online ISBN 978-1-83769-672-7
eBook (PDF) ISBN 978-1-83769-674-1

Meet the editors

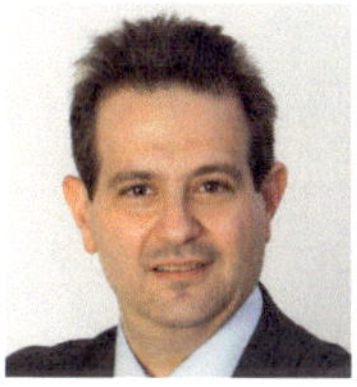

Dr. Dimitrios D. Nikolopoulos is a graduate of Athens University Medical School. He specialized in orthopaedic surgery and traumatology at the Orthopaedic Clinic of the General Hospital "Asklepeion Voulas," Greece, where he focused on sports injuries and foot pathology. He also specialized in hand surgery at the Microsurgery Clinic, KAT Hospital, Greece. He trained in arthroscopic restoration of hip pathology alongside Dr. Alexis Nogier at the Clinic Maussins-Nollet, Paris, and has continued his training in arthroscopic rehabilitation of sports injuries of the knee, shoulder, and ankle as well as the treatment and surgical correction of foot disorders. Dr. Nikolopoulos has published forty-two original journal articles on knee (valgus knee) and shoulder surgery (arthroscopic and minimally invasive new techniques), osteoporotic spine and hip fractures, and in vitro research on bone and cartilage metabolism. He has also presented more than 180 oral and poster presentations internationally within the last decade, namely on sports injury of the knee, shoulder, and ankle joints and arthritis of the knee and hip. He is a doctor of the University of Athens and a member of the Greek Traumatology and Orthopaedic Society, Greek Arthroscopy Society, European Arthroscopy Association, and European Society of Sports Traumatology, Knee Surgery and Arthroscopy (ESSKA), among others.

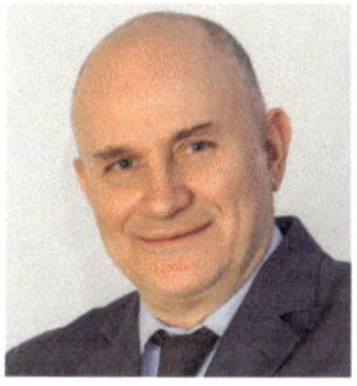

Dr. George K. Safos, MD, specializes in orthopaedic surgery and traumatology with an interest in sports medicine (knee, hip, ankle, elbow, and shoulder arthroscopic surgery) as well as total hip and knee replacement surgery. As a well-published doctor, he now serves as a medical orthopaedic consultant and the primary doctor to various athletic teams, dance groups, and foreign diplomatic missions. He is a graduate of Athens University Medical School and completed his residency in orthopaedic surgery and traumatology at the General Hospital "Asklepeion Voulas," Greece. He then completed two fellowships in the United States at the National Institutes of Health (NIH) and the University of Miami. Dr. Safos also obtained a post-graduate degree in tissue banking at the National University of Singapore with a United Nations scholarship.

Contents

Preface

The number of cases of shoulder pathology and disorders has been increasing in the last three decades due to various reasons. One reason for the increased prevalence of shoulder injuries is trauma, which can occur at work or due to vehicular accidents, among other reasons. Another reason for increased injuries is overuse of the joint, such as occurs in demanding sports and hobbies like basketball, volleyball, skiing, and so on.

Shoulder Surgery – Open vs Arthroscopic Techniques presents a comprehensive overview of current research and clinical expertise for orthopedic surgeons and other professionals involved with the assessment, management, and rehabilitation of shoulder pathology.

This book is a concise and up-to-date resource on common shoulder disorders and therapeutic solutions, conservative or operative, with open or arthroscopic techniques. It discusses the most common shoulder conditions, such as those caused by trauma, fractures, instability, and so on, as well as their pathology, evaluation, and management. In each chapter, the reader will learn about anatomy and biomechanical changes in the function of the shoulder joint due to the specific pathology, along with symptoms and clinical evaluation tests, radiological imaging, and other investigations secondly needed, as well as principles of non-surgical and surgical management of the shoulder pathology.

This book is a team project, edited by two renowned researchers and clinicians, and shoulder surgeons Dr. Nikolopoulos Dimitrios and Dr. George Safos. The five contributing authors include prominent clinical experts and researchers, orthopedic surgeons with expertise in shoulder surgery and arthroscopy, and physiotherapists.

The following sections discuss the chapters' contents.

1. Instability: Open vs. Arthroscopic

The shoulder joint is the most dislocated major joint, with a reported incidence of ~2%. About 95% of shoulder dislocations are traumatic, while the other 5% are due to predisposing factors such as generalized ligamentous laxity. Most (90%) shoulder dislocations are anterior from direct force on the arm in the "ABER" position (Abduction- External Rotation), and the rest (10%) are posterior. Symptomatic instability following dislocation is common, especially in young and active patients. Recurrent instability occurs in 50%–96% of patients whose first dislocation occurred when they were younger than 20 years, and in 40%–74% of patients whose first dislocation occurred between the ages of 20 and 40 years [1–4]. Operative treatment reduces the risk of recurrence, mainly in young athletes. Several studies in the last decade have compared arthroscopic and open shoulder instability repair techniques.

In the case of traumatic shoulder dislocation in the younger population or competitive sport players, accompanied by bone injury on CTs or MRIs (Bony Bankart or Hill-Sachs), surgical treatment is recommended as soon as possible to avoid recurring dislocation and further joint damage. Proponents of the open technique have debated that the open procedure allows for a more anatomic and secure repair with improved anchor orientation, whereas proponents of the arthroscopic technique have opposed that arthroscopy avoids the complications associated with open approaches, such as infection, violation of the subscapularis, and arthrofibrosis, while providing an equivalent repair with a faster recovery [3–4]. The classic open Bankart procedure includes an incision of the subscapularis tendon and capsule to expose the anterior aspect of the labrum and capsule for secure reattachment to the glenoid rim with suture passed through bone tunnels. Multiple variations have been used to expose the joint, to repair the ligaments, and to treat associated capsular laxity. Arthroscopic stabilization for recurrent anterior instability has undergone significant changes over the last two decades. Nowadays, this is the method preferred by most shoulder surgeons. There are several retrospective comparative trials, case-control studies, randomized controlled trials, and meta-analyses comparing both techniques with contradictory results [1–5]. This chapter conducts a literature review comparing open versus arthroscopic procedures, assessing failure rates, complications, return to activity, costs, and hospital stays.

2. Glenoid Bone Defect in Anterior Shoulder Instability

As analyzed in Chapter 2, anterior shoulder instability is a common orthopedic situation that often affects the glenohumeral joint's bony architecture as well as the capsulolabral complex [6]. Recurrent anterior shoulder instability may result from a spectrum of overlapping, often coexistent factors, one of which is glenoid bone loss. Nevertheless, patients with recurrent shoulder dislocations are at increased risk for glenohumeral bone loss. That's because each instability event leads firstly to the accumulation of additional glenoid and secondly to humeral head bone defects [7, 8]. The Hill-Sachs lesion is an osseous defect of the humeral head that is typically associated with anterior shoulder instability. Several classification systems have been recommended for glenohumeral bone loss. Thorough evaluation of bone loss preoperatively, in terms of location, size, and significance, is essential, for successful treatment. Furthermore, apart from the degree of bone loss, effective treatment also means reconstruction of the injured soft-tissue structures (labrum, capsule, glenohumeral ligaments, and rotator cuff). Numerous imaging modalities have been proposed, including shoulder CT and three-dimensional reconstruction, and shoulder MRI. Three-dimensional imaging has proven particularly useful in preoperative planning to evaluate glenoid and humeral defects. Different arthroscopic repair techniques, open Bankart procedure, capsular plication, remplissage, Latarjet technique, iliac crest, and other bone grafts for augmentation, along with post-operative rehabilitation, offer the surgeon different treatment options according to the type of lesion [7–9]. This chapter analyzes the clinical symptoms, imaging evaluation, and therapeutic procedures for anterior shoulder instability. Nonsurgical management, including focused rehabilitation, is acceptable in cases of small bony defects and patients older than 60 years. Surgical options include arthroscopic and open techniques for unstable cases or young adults and athletic patients.

3. **Arthroscopic Assisted versus Open Reduction and Internal Fixation of Greater Tuberosity Fractures of the Proximal Humerus**

Isolated greater tuberosity fractures account for up to a fifth of all proximal humeral fractures. Several retrospective cohort studies and case series outcomes have been reported after treatment of the greater tuberosity fractures of the proximal humerus [10–14]. As the greater tuberosity is the insertion site mainly of the posterior superior rotator cuff, fractures can have a significant impact on shoulder functional outcomes [12]. Thorough patient evaluation is required to make an appropriate diagnosis of these fractures and choose the proper treatment. Usually, surgical management is considered when there is displacement of 5 mm or greater of the fragmented parts. Although the reduction of displaced greater tuberosity fractures has traditionally been performed with open techniques, arthroscopic techniques are now available [12–14]. The most reliable techniques of fixation of the greater tuberosity incorporate the rotator cuff tendon-bone junction rather than direct bone-to-bone fixation [13, 14]. This chapter analyzes the isolated greater tuberosity fractures of the proximal humerus and discusses important aspects of the epidemiology, anatomy, fracture classification, associated injuries, and treatment procedures. The authors use their experience and review recent literature on evaluating diagnostic criteria and treatment outcomes (open vs arthroscopic).

4. **Arthroscopic Tenotomy versus Open Tenodesis of the Long Head Biceps Brachii Tendon**

Some of the major causes of shoulder pain and dysfunction are lesions of the proximal long head of the biceps tendon (LHB). The role of the LHB in causing pain has been a source of controversy for many years, and extensive literature is available discussing anatomy, function, pathology, and, most importantly, appropriate treatment. In most cases, conservative management is preferred, which includes rest, nonsteroidal anti-inflammatory medicines, physical therapy, and steroid injections. Surgery is frequently recommended if symptoms that have been treated conservatively for more than three months continue. Surgical treatment of the LHB is also recommended in cases of isolated symptomatic pathology, such as SLAP II (or higher stages of Snyder classification), partial tears, hour-glass deformity, or in concomitant rotator cuff lesions with biceps instability and tendinitis and finally at the time of shoulder arthroplasty. Despite this, there is a lack of consensus in the literature regarding the management of biceps-related pathology. Biceps tenotomy and tenodesis are common surgical treatment options when dealing with LHB-related pathology. This chapter discusses surgical options (open versus arthroscopic) with a focus on the different options for biceps tenodesis. It also discusses outcomes and complications [14, 15].

5. **Assessment of Upper Trapezium Pain and Muscle Strength after Posiconal Release and Myofascial Release**

Trapezius myalgia (TM) is pain, stiffness, and tightness of the upper trapezius muscle. It is characterized by acute or persistent neck–shoulder pain. TM, which can last a few days or longer, is not a health disorder or disease but rather a symptom of an existing underlying condition [16]. The trapezius is a large fan-shaped muscle that extends from the cervical to the thoracic region on the posterior aspect of the cervical and upper thoracic spine and attaches onto the clavicle and scapula. It consists of three parts with different actions: (1) the superior fibers of the trapezius, which elevate the shoulder girdle, (2) the middle fibers of the trapezius, which retract the scapula, and (3) the inferior fibers of the trapezius, which depress the scapula. Typically, pain occurs in the superior fibers of the trapezius in TM [16, 17]. The most typical symptoms of TM are sudden onset of pain in the upper trapezius, muscle stiffness and spasms, tightness of the neck–shoulder complex, heaviness of the head and occipital headache, and tenderness of the upper trapezius area. Some other less common symptoms are low mood, anxiety, and paresthesia [17]. In general, no objective diagnostic methods are available specifically for TM. The diagnosis is mostly based on symptom presentation and history of illness. Thorough subjective and objective assessment, including neurological exam and shoulder evaluation, should be performed. Imaging studies, such as MRIs of the cervical and thoracic part of the spine, for evaluating a possible disc hernia or other pathologies can be useful if there is no improvement in symptoms or when neurological symptoms exist or if red flags present. Furthermore, diagnostic injections may be useful. Different forms of exercise are recommended for acute or persistent neck pain [18]. Physical activity and exercise have been proven to give the most immediate and long-term pain relief in patients with TM. Both general fitness training and specific strength training generate significant effects on decreasing pain; however, strength training has been proven to be more effective [18]. Following a specific neck strengthening exercise program for up to one year can lead to long-term reduction and further prevention of recurring pain even after the strength program has ceased [17–18]. In this chapter, the authors discuss their experience and outcomes for upper trapezium pain and muscle strength after positional and myofascial release.

This book offers up-to-date coverage of shoulder function and dysfunction as well as discusses practical approaches for patient evaluation and treatment alternatives, including open and arthroscopic procedures and surgical and nonsurgical techniques. Furthermore, it provides a balanced view of both open and arthroscopic techniques so the treating professional can choose the right procedures for their patients.

Dr. Dimitrios D. Nikolopoulos and Dr. George K. Safos (MD)
Orthopaedic Surgeon, Arthroscopist,
Central Clinic of Athens,
Athens, Greece

References

[1] Hurley ET, Davey MS, Montgomery C, O'Doherty R, Gaafar M, Pauzenberger L, et al. Arthroscopic bankart repair versus open Latarjet for recurrent shoulder instability in athletes. Orthopaedic Journal of Sports Medicine. 8 Sep 2021;**9**(9):23259671211023801. DOI: 10.1177/23259671211023801

[2] Hurley ET, Toale JP, Davey MS, Colasanti CA, Pauzenberger L, Strauss EJ, et al. Remplissage for anterior shoulder instability with Hill-Sachs lesions: A systematic review and meta-analysis. Journal of Shoulder and Elbow Surgery. 2020;**29**(12):2487-2494. DOI: 10.1016/j.jse.2020.06.021

[3] Hurley ET, Fat DL, Farrington SK, Mullett H. Open versus arthroscopic Latarjet procedure for anterior shoulder instability: A systematic review and meta-analysis. The American Journal of Sports Medicine. 2019;**47**(5):1248-1253. DOI: 10.1177/0363546518759540

[4] Huerta A, Rincón G, Peidro L, Combalia A, Sastre S. Controversies in the surgical management of shoulder instability: Open vs arthroscopic procedures. The Open Orthopaedics Journal. 2017;**31**(11):875-881. DOI: 10.2174/1874325001711010875

[5] Provencher MT, Frank RM, Leclere LE, Metzger PD, Ryu JJ, Bernhardson A, et al. The Hill-Sachs lesion: Diagnosis, classification, and management. J Am Acad Orthop Surg. 2012;**20**(4):242-52. doi: 10.5435/JAAOS-20-04-242

[6] Eric C Makhni 1, Joseph S Tramer, Matthew J J Anderson, William N Levine. Evaluating Bone Loss in Anterior Shoulder Instability. Journal of the American Academy of Orthopaedic Surgeons. 2022;**30**(12):563-572. DOI: 10.5435/JAAOS-D-22-00016

[7] Moya D, Aydin N, Yamamoto N, Simone JP, Robles PP, Tytherleigh-Strong G, et al. Current concepts in anterior glenohumeral instability: Diagnosis and treatment. SICOT Journal. 2021;**7**:48. DOI: 10.1051/sicotj/2021048

[8] Piaseck DP, Verma NN, Romeo AA, Levine WN, Bach Jr BR, Provencher MT. Glenoid bone deficiency in recurrent anterior shoulder instability: Diagnosis and management. Journals of the American Academy of Orthopaedic Surgeons. 2009;**17**(8):482-493. DOI: 10.5435/00124635-200908000-00002

[9] Rabinowitz J, Friedman R, Eichinger JK. Management of glenoid bone loss with anterior shoulder instability: Indications and outcomes. Current Reviews in Musculoskeletal Medicine. 2017;**10**(4):452-462. DOI: 10.1007/s12178-017-9439-y

[10] DeBottis D, Anavian J, Green A. Surgical management of isolated greater tuberosity fractures of the proximal humerus. Orthopedic Clinics of North America. 2014;**45**(2):207-218. DOI: 10.1016/j.ocl.2013.12.007

[11] Green A, Izzi Jr J. Isolated fractures of the greater tuberosity of the proximal humerus. Journal of Shoulder and Elbow Surgery. 2003;**12**(6):641-649. DOI: 10.1016/s1058-2746(02)86811-2

[12] Miltenberg B, Masood R, Katsiaunis A, Moverman MA, Puzzitiello RN, Pagani NR, et al. Fracture dislocations of the proximal humerus treated with open reduction and internal fixation: A systematic

review. Journal of Shoulder and Elbow Surgery. 2022;**31**(10):e480-e489. DOI: 10.1016/j.jse.2022.04.018

[13] Huntley SR, Lehtonen EJ, Robin JX, Arguello AM, Rouleau DM, Brabston EW, et al. Outcomes of surgical fixation of greater tuberosity fractures: A systematic review. Orthopaedics and Traumatology: Surgery and Research. 2020;**106**(6):1119-1126. DOI: 10.1016/j.otsr.2020.05.005

[14] AlQahtani SM, Bicknell RT. Outcomes following long head of biceps tendon tenodesis. Current Reviews in Musculoskeletal Medicine. Dec 2016;**9**(4):378-387. DOI: 10.1007/s12178-016-9362-7. PMID: 27599831; PMCID: PMC5127942

[15] Slenker NR, Lawson K, Ciccotti MG, Dodson CC, Cohen SB. Biceps tenotomy versus tenodesis: Clinical outcomes. Arthroscopy. 2012;**28**:576-582. DOI: 10.1016/j.arthro.2011.10.017. PMID: 22284407

[16] Meulemeester K, Calders P, De Pauw R, Grymonpon I, Govaerts A, Cagnie B. Morphological and physiological differences in the upper trapezius muscle in patients with work-related trapezius myalgia compared to healthy controls: A systematic review. Musculoskeletal Science and Practice. 2017;**29**:43-51

[17] Waling K, Sundelin G, Ahlgren C, Järvholm B. Perceived pain before and after three exercise programs – A controlled clinical trial of women with work-related trapezius myalgia. Pain. 2000;**85**(1-2):201-207. DOI: 10.1016/s0304-3959(99)00265-1

[18] Irene J, Karin HR. Strategies for prevention and management of musculoskeletal conditions. Neck pain. Best Practice and Research Clinical Rheumatology. 2007;**21**(1):93-108

Chapter 1

Instability: Open vs. Arthroscopic

Adrián Aziz Cortés de la Fuente
and Maximiliano Cruz Palacios

Abstract

Anterior shoulder instability is common among young and active individuals, and anterior instability is the most common in 80.3% of cases, which may be the result of trauma or laxity. The glenohumeral joint is the most mobile joint of the human body, formed by the humeral head and the glenoid surface of the scapula, and its stability is given by static and dynamic stabilizers. Typically, a detailed interrogation and an accurate physical examination are required to diagnose and determine the source of the instability. Of great importance is the performance of provocative tests within our physical examination. These are done intentionally to reproduce the symptoms of instability. For treatment options, there is no universal standardized criterion; however, there are different tools such as ISIS and patient-dependent factors, which help us to make better decisions and use the best therapeutic tool, always looking at the type of patient we have in front of us. The conclusion is that different open or closed therapeutic techniques can be used for the management of anterior shoulder instability with similar success and recurrence rates.

Keywords: instability, Bankart, Dass, Latarjet, shoulder, arthroscopy

1. Introduction

Glenohumeral instability is a common problem in young, active individuals with high functional demands on the shoulder. It occurs in a wide range of patients who need different individualized treatment strategies. Anterior instability is the most common at 80.3%, followed by posterior (10.3%) and multidirectional (9.4%). However, many aspects of the management of these injuries are controversial and much of this is due to a lack of strong evidence in guiding treatment [1, 2].

Shoulder instability results from trauma, microtrauma, and a history of joint hypermobility due to laxity. Traumatic anterior instability is associated with some soft tissue injury and the typical Bankart injury with or without capsular laxity. Soft tissue repair has been shown to have high success rates, either open or arthroscopic. In very rare cases, bony injuries are associated with recurrent instability. There is a guideline in the literature regarding the surgical treatment of anterior shoulder instability with significant glenoid bone loss. Options include Latarjet or Bristow procedures and bone graft blocks. Procedures that transfer the coracoid have been shown to carry an increased risk of loss of mobility, development of osteoarthritis, screw fatigue, and resorption or nonunion of the graft [3].

The diagnosis of anterior instability requires clinical evaluation, determining the patient's risk for recurrent instability, and thus dictating appropriate treatment. Similarly, the choice of imaging studies needed in the study of anterior instability continues to be variable due to the lack of standardized guidelines [1].

The purpose of this chapter is to present a broad overview of the anatomy, biomechanics, pathophysiology, diagnostic process, non-operative management, and surgical management of glenohumeral joint instability.

2. Anatomy

The glenohumeral joint has the greatest mobility of any joint in the human body, as well as the greatest predisposition for dislocation. It is distributed into three joints: glenohumeral, acromioclavicular, and sternoclavicular. These last two, in combination with the spaces between the scapula and the thorax, are known as the scapulothoracic joint. The three diarthrodial joints are constituted with little bony stability and the stability relies on their ligaments and the adjacent muscles of the glenohumeral joint [4].

2.1 Glenohumeral joint

Formed by the head of the humerus and the glenoid surface of the scapula, the long, spherical head articulates against a small glenoid fossa, a relationship comparable to a golf ball in support. Stability of this ball is provided by dynamic and static stabilizers acting across the joint [4].

The humeral head is long, globular, and one-third of the sphere articulates with the glenoid. The head tilts 130 to 150 degrees relative to the diaphysis. The vertical dimension of the articular portion is about 48 mm, with a radius of curvature of 25 mm; the transverse dimension is 45 mm, with a radius of curvature of 22 mm. The bicipital groove is 30 degrees medial to the axis of the humeral diaphysis. The greater tuberosity is part of the lateral wall, and the lesser tuberosity is part of the medial wall of the bicipital groove [4].

The glenoid cavity has the shape of an inverted comma; in the uppermost area is the tail, it is narrow, and the lower portion is wider. The transversal line that divides these two surfaces corresponds to the epiphyseal line of the glenoid cavity. The glenoid has an articular surface covered by hyaline cartilage. In its center is a circular area where the cartilage is thinned. This area, according to DePalma, is related to the region of greatest contact with the humerus [4].

The vertical dimension of the glenoid is 35 mm, and the transverse diameter is 25 mm. Saha noted that the glenoid position can be retroverted or anteverted with respect to the plane of the scapula. Approximately 75% of the shoulders studied had retroversion of 7.4 degrees and the remaining 25% had an anteversion of 2 to 10 degrees. The superior portion of a line drawn from superior to inferior is angled on average about 15 degrees medial to the scapular plane. Based on the contact surface, Saha et al. originally classified the glenohumeral joint into three types. In type A, the humeral surface has a smaller radius of coverage than the glenoid. In type B, the humerus and glenoid have similar areas of coverage and a larger area of contact. In type C, the humeral surface has a larger radius of curvature than the glenoid, and the contact between these two surfaces is limited to the periphery. However, Soslowsky

DOI: http://dx.doi.org/10.5772/intechopen.1002635

found that the humeral head-to-glenoid ratio is 3.12:1 and 2.0:1 for males and females, respectively [4].

Thus, these authors attributed the relative instability of the shoulder not to shape or incongruity, but to the small surface area of the glenoid compared to the humerus [4].

2.2 Glenohumeral ligaments

The glenohumeral ligaments are reinforcements of the joint capsule. Their functions depend on the integrity of the collagen, their insertion site, and the position of the arm in space [4].

2.2.1 Superior glenohumeral ligament

A constant structure is present in 97% of the shoulders examined in DePalma's classic study of anatomy. Three anatomical variants can be found at its glenoid insertion:

1. It may initiate from a common origin with the biceps tendon.

2. It may originate from the labrum.

3. It may originate with the medial glenohumeral ligament.

Its insertion is at the fovea capitis and lies just superior to the lesser tuberosity. The size and integrity of the ligament is variable. Biomechanical studies this ligament contributing very little to the static stability of the glenohumeral joint. Its relative contribution is contingent on the integrity and thickness of the collagen fibers [4].

2.2.2 Middle glenohumeral ligament

It is the ligament with the greatest variation in size of all glenohumeral ligaments. It has been shown in different studies to be absent in 27% of specimen studies [4].

When present, it originates from the labrum below the superior glenohumeral ligament or from the glenoid neck. It inserts into the humerus medial to the lesser tuberosity, behind the tendon of the subscapularis muscle to which it is attached [5]. Another variation, the tendon is attached to the anterior portion of the capsule. When it is thick enough, it provides anterior restriction to humeral translation [4].

2.2.3 Inferior glenohumeral ligament

This ligament is a structural complex, which is the main static stabilizer at shoulder abduction. It is a hammock-like structure that originates from the glenoid and inserts into the anatomical neck of the humerus, and consists of an anterior band, a posterior band, and an axillary recess, which lies between the two [4].

The origins of the anterior and posterior bands on the glenoid are in terms of the face of a clock. The anterior band originated from between the 2 o'clock and 4 o'clock positions and the posterior band from between the 7 o'clock and 9 o'clock positions.

On the humeral head side, it inserts in an approximately 90-degree arc just below the articular margin of the humeral head [4].

Considering that this ligament has a hammock function to support the humeral head provides the basis for explaining how damage to one of its portions can affect the opposite side. This concept has clinical significance for the treatment of instability [4].

3. Clinical history

Clinicians evaluating patients with acute and chronic instability should obtain a detailed clinical history documented in detail to recognize a patient with a first-time dislocation or a chronic dislocator [3]. This includes the following elements:

3.1 First occasion dislocated patients

- After an acute event, they will typically report a history of recent high-energy trauma that is the cause of the dislocation.

- Clinicians should of the following aspects: degree of trauma (high or low energy), degree of athletic activity and position and discern between true dislocation events [3].

3.2 In patients with chronic dislocation

This typically occurs after decreased range of motion with significant impact on activities of daily living.

- The initial injury is overlooked, and the patient develops chronic and recurrent instability.

- Clinical suspicion is warranted in the presence of the following: a history of epilepsy or electric shock and polytrauma, where instability may have gone unnoticed [3].

- Low energy, recurrent subluxation cases: Episodes of shoulder instability during sleep should indicate a more complex instability, which means bone loss [3].

4. Physical examination

Because of the complex, multifaceted role of the shoulder, it is an important and common source of pathology, as we have seen especially in athletes. As with any examination, a detailed questioning can be of great help. To locate shoulder pathology, the interview should begin by identifying the possible causes of the symptomatology. In case of trauma, the location of the trauma (anterior or posterior) should be questioned, and any functional restriction should be identified. The patient's age should be of importance; certain pathologies, such as rotator cuff injuries and impingement syndrome, should sometimes be ruled out because of the patient's age. A history of previous trauma should be suspected of instability, and the presence of neurological disorders may increase the risk of various pathologies [6].

Examination should follow a pattern and begins with inspection, and proceeds with palpation, active and passive ranges of motion, strength, and neurological examination. A very important component of the physical examination is the ranges of motion; normal includes elevation 150 to 180 degrees, extension 40 to 60 degrees, abduction 150 to 180 degrees, external rotation 60 to 90 degrees, and internal rotation 50 to 70 degrees [6].

Particularly in athletes, where overhead throwing or overhead activities are performed, such as baseball pitchers, evaluation of the glenohumeral labrum is essential. The speed test can help identify anterior shoulder pathology, as well as injury to the insertion of the long head of the biceps. The most sensitive and specific test for labral pathology is the O'Brien test, which is performed by passively flexing the patient's arm to 90 degrees and adducting it 10 degrees. The forearm with the hand is brought into pronation, and the arm is internally rotated until the thumb points toward the floor. This position is held against resistance, positive with pain or weakness. For the second part of this test, the arm is externally rotated, or the forearm is supinated so that the thumb is directed upward, and again forced downward against patient resistance [7]. Reduced discomfort on change of thumb position suggests a labral lesion [6].

Examination of instability should begin with a purposeful search for ligament laxity of the patient. Joint laxity, or a Beighton score, should be taken when evaluating ligament instability [6].

4.1 Provocation maneuvers

4.1.1 Anterior apprehension test

This maneuver is performed by lying the patient supine on the examination table. Place the shoulder at 90 degrees of abduction and 90 degrees of external rotation while applying an anterior force to the proximal humerus. The test is positive if it reproduces the symptoms of the anterior instability [3].

The apprehension test in low degrees of abduction may suggest glenoid bone loss. The clinician can determine if the apprehension position triggers the patient's feelings of anterior instability [3].

4.1.2 Jobe repositioning test

It is used with a prior apprehension maneuver. Once the patient reports subjective feeling, the examiner applies force posteriorly directly while holding the shoulder in the same apprehension position. A resolution or improvement of symptoms indicates a positive test [3].

4.1.3 Load and shift test

The examiner uses one hand to apply axial load through the elbow toward the center of the humeral head and pressing on the glenoid. Direct forces are applied anteriorly or posteriorly to or –46 degrees and 90 degrees of shoulder abduction. An increase in translation with increasing degrees of abduction implies inferior glenohumeral ligament involvement [3].

It can be graded as follows:

- Grade 1: Increased translation compared to the normal shoulder.
- Grade 2: Increased translation of the humeral head, but no more, to the glenoid rim.
- Grade 3: Indicates a translation of the humeral head over the glenoid rim.

5. Treatment options

Dislocation rate is 0.08 per 1000 people annually, and anterior dislocation accounts for 80%. In younger patients under 25 the risk of recurrence is high as 95% as reported by Rowe.

Boileau and Balg, ISIS score may be a guidance to bony augmentation beyond a soft tissue alone procedure utilizing the threshold of 6 to do a Latarjet, and other authors have suggested lowering it [8–13].

It was described by Sugaya et al. that the dislocation in anterior direction of the humeral head accompanied the lesion presenting an avulsion of the inferior glenohumeral ligament in 97%, bony lesion and/or HAGL in 50 and 9%, respectively, like the example in **Figure 1** [8, 10].

In first-time dislocators, the treatment of choice could be conservative depending on ISIS and other specific related patient factors, and on the other hand in recurrence >2 dislocations, the gold standard of treatment could be an arthroscopic Bankart; this technique was first described by Arthur Sidney Blundell Bankart in 1923, at that time, other techniques were used, the Clairmont and Ehrlich, Nicola, and the Handerson sling operations. The original technique was published in the British Medical Journal, an open technique with wide exposure of the anterior glenoid rim and utilizing a coracoid osteotomy and subscapularis tenotomy, then suturing the capsule-labral

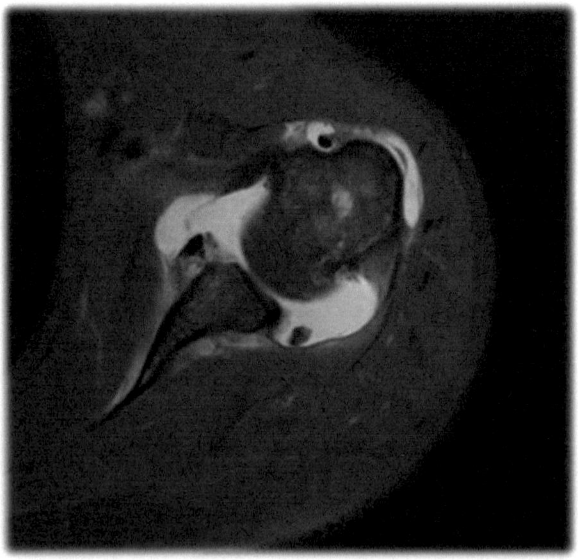

Figure 1.
MRI T2 axial view showing a bony Bankart lesion.

injury. In contrast, the modern arthroscopic Bankart described by Dr. Peter Millett is accomplished with the knowledge of other concomitant pathologies that can be treated at the same time but with the same principles using 3 to 4 portals.

So we need to think about the pitfalls of the technique for doing only a Bankart repair like in the present case in **Figure 1**, considering the extent of the glenoid bone loss, visualizing associated ALPS, HAGL, the use of less than three suture anchors, inadequate mobilization of the capsule-labral tissues, inadequate plication, and placement of the anchors to medial of the glenoid. With this in mind, we can say that Bankart repair is still the treatment of choice being the arthroscopic technique with its variations the gold standard [8, 14].

Glenoid bone loss increases the contact pressure by 300% in defects of more than 30%, and this was described as "inverted pear" shape of the glenoid, which has been considered a risk factor for arthroscopic stabilization [8, 13].

Conservative treatment has shown recurrences of 58% with end stage arthritis to 39% in cases of recurrent instability [7, 9, 13, 15].

Losses of less than 20–25% are associated with recurrences as 19% in soft tissue-only techniques in cases where there is more than 25% recurrence up to 67% [8, 9, 16].

Augmentation procedures must be considered in patients like in **Figure 2**, Latarjet is the gold standard in defined critical GBL of >25%, but as we previously mentioned all associated pathology as Hill-Sachs lesions must be taken into account present in 65–67% of the first event and 84–93% in recurrent cases (**Figure 3**) [8, 17]. Computed tomography with 3D reconstruction of a patient with critical bone loss.

We follow the recommendation by Di Giacommo were an "on track" Hill-Sachs lesion with GBL of >20% requiring augmentation procedures such as Bristow, Latarjet, the use of autologous iliac crest, femoral head, distal tibia, and clavicle grafts for augmentation and "off-track" HS with glenoid loss of more than 20%. Are amenable for a Latarjet [9, 10, 13, 18, 19].

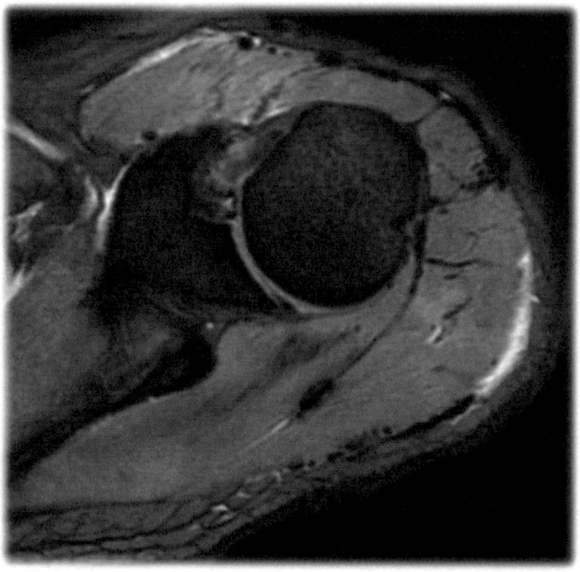

Figure 2.
MRI T2 axial image of a right shoulder with a Bankart lesion.

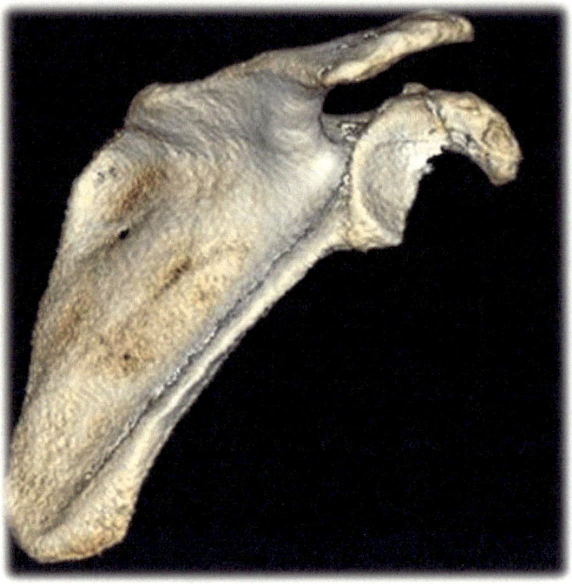

Figure 3.
3D CT scan showing critical bone loss of a right shoulder.

Isolated arthroscopic Bankart procedure reports recurrences 28.4% vs. 3% in Latarjet, so there has been an interest in performing this procedure in a primary way for all cases of anterior recurrent pathology with high-risk patients with ISIS >4 and in revision cases.

The complication rates with the gold standard treatment are: 30% being neurovascular injury, 1.8% recurrent instability, and infection in 6%. In cases of failed Latarjet, GBL is difficult to manage with recurrences of up to 12% after an Eden-Hybinette procedure reporting 33% of poor results [5, 11, 15, 20].

Moreover, moderate-to-severe osteoarthritis has been reported in 18% of patients without recurrence and up to 26% in patients treated with Latarjet surgical stabilization [7].

The Eden-Hybinette procedure with autologous iliac crest graft has shown good results with lower recurrent rates of instability, the present indication for this technique includes severe glenoid bone loss of more than 40%, recurrent instability after a Latarjet or distal tibia graft, but the main problem of this technique is the morbidity of the donor site and the accelerated rate for postoperative glenohumeral arthritis in up to 20% [21, 22]. Taverna et al. described an arthroscopic technique in 26 patients, reporting 88.5% satisfaction without recurrent dislocations and graft integration of 92.3% [21].

In the Eden-Hybinette procedure, 17.6% of complications have been described, compared to 17.2% in arthroscopic Latarjet and Bristow-Latarjet in 15% [20].

Last but not least, a novel technique based on the transfer of the long head of the biceps called "dynamic anterior stabilization" must be discussed since, although in general, arthroscopic Bankart continues to be the gold standard, the variety and severity of the lesions shared in the pathology of anterior instability, be it bone loss, Hill-Sachs, hyperlaxity, quality of the tissue, and so this being the case when the treatment becomes more complex, the choice of the gestures coupled with the repair becomes confusing.

In addition to the concern for reducing the rate of complications to which the gold standard of instability with subcritical bone loss has led, the Latarjet compared to the Bankart plus remplissage has shown improvement in the reduction of recurrence of 7% vs. 9.8% but with an increase in complications of 9% vs. 1%, respectively [23].

The oldest antecedent of this procedure dates from a labrumplasty described in 1967 called the Vainstein procedure, but in 2018 Collin and Ladermann describe the transposition of the head of the long head of the biceps through the subscapularis and to the anterior glenoid rim by tunneling it for what is considered an inlay technique performing fixation with an interference screw and subsequently with a suspension system. Immediately afterward in 2019 [24], Toussaint describes a modification of the technique to an onlay in which they performed an augmentation of the labrum by inserting the tendon into the glenoid rim.

In both techniques, the long head tendon is prepared outside, so it is not a totally arthroscopic technique [24, 25].

In 2021, results were published in 22 patients with a subcritical bone loss of <20% in which they had a 13.6% recurrence rate which happened in the first patients and could be related to the learning curve [26].

In the same year, Campos and Angelo describe their onlay arthroscopic technique in which they perform a double-row all-suture anchor fixation to the anterior glenoid rim using only three portals. They presented 18 patients with bone loss of less than 20% and follow-up of 48 months; without recurrences in the subgroup analysis of patients without hyperlaxity, WOSI and Rowe scales improved significantly and without complications [27, 28].

Regarding the biomechanics of DAAS, various studies have been carried out, which demonstrate the sling and hammock effect, with decreases of anterior translation, and without a decrease in external rotation compared to Bankart repair in bone losses of 10–20%; additionally in losses of less than 13% it is significantly stronger than the Bankart at 16.3 and 16.6% against the conjoint tendon.

To mention other advantages, it is possible to manage the SLAP lesion in the same procedure, hardware is not handled, and as previously mentioned, neurovascular complications are reduced, the disadvantage would be returning to sports at 6 months compared to 3 months for the Latarjet [28–30].

6. Open vs. arthroscopic treatment

Recurrent shoulder instability results in decreased performance in sports and certain demanding military activities. Bankart's lesion is present in 85–90% of cases of traumatic shoulder dislocations. The age and activity level of the patient who suffers an acute dislocation best correlates with the risk of recurrence after medical treatment [31].

The open Bankart repair allows the ability to perform open capsular plication. The use of arthroscopic stabilization in chronic anterior instability was initially reported to have a lower success rate than open surgery (**Figure 4**). However, with advances in arthroscopic instrumentation and techniques, results continue to improve [31]. Numerous studies with 2-year follow-up have demonstrated comparable efficacy between open and arthroscopic techniques [32, 33].

Indications.

arthroscopic procedures	open procedures
• Glenoid Bone Loss from 0 to 10% • Preserve external rotation. • Glenoid Bone Loss with good soft tissue quality	• Glenoid defects greater than 20% • Youth, male, participation in contact sports

Figure 4.
Arthroscopic indications.

Bottoni et al. found a long-term failure rate of 14.3% for arthroscopic surgeries and 12.5% for open surgeries. Subjective outcome tests between the two treatment groups were similar at 32-month follow-up and 15-year follow-up. The value on the UCLA marker postoperatively was 31.4 at 12 months and 28.6 at 15 years. There was no statistically significant difference between treatments in all functional tests measured at 15-year postoperative follow-up ($p > 0.05$) [31]. Long-term follow-up results agree that there is no difference in failure rates between arthroscopic and open techniques [18]. Burkhart and De Beer reported inferior results with an arthroscopic technique in the context of Hill-Sachs hooking lesions and suggested reconstruction with an alternative technique, especially if associated with critical glenoid bone loss [19]. However, in this study there were only three patients with this type of defect and follow-up was limited to 27 months. In conclusions, open or arthroscopic Bankart repairs are safe and reproducible in returning most patients to their pre-injury activity status. In the context of an off-track injury, there are higher failure rates regardless of the technique used [31].

In terms of Latarjet surgery it is a procedure that regardless of whether the arthroscopic or open technique is used has reported high success rates (**Figure** 5). The Laterjet procedure is a well-established treatment option with favorable long-term results. Re-luxation rates following this procedure are estimated to be around 4-5% [34].

Lafosse et al. proposed that the arthroscopic technique offers advantages of more accurate graft placement, faster recovery, decreased stiffness, and cosmetic benefits [35].

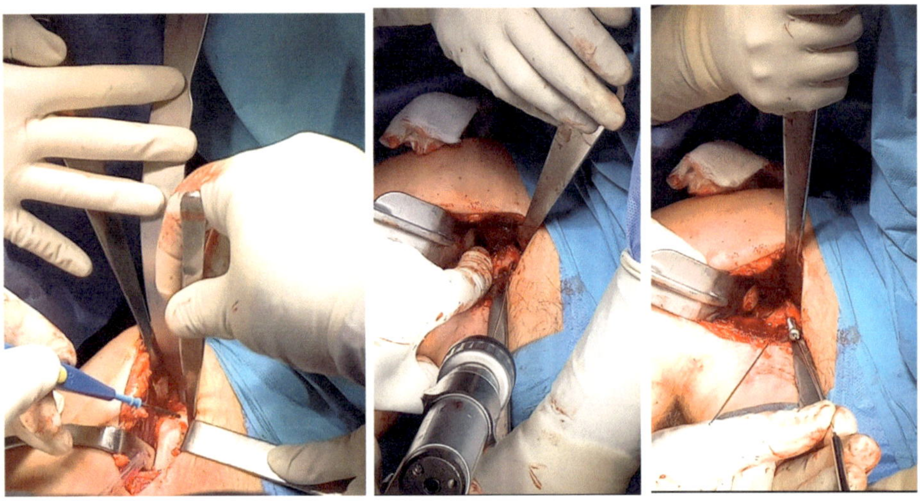

Figure 5.
Latarjet procedure, open technique.

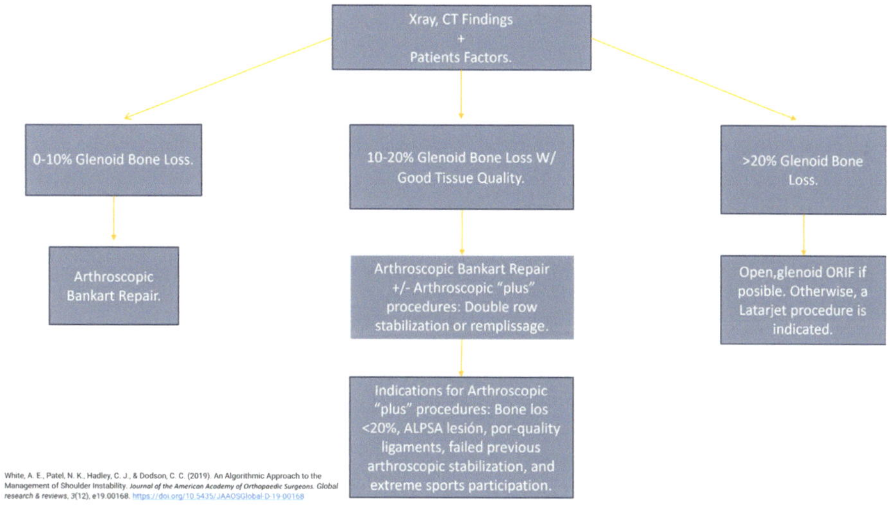

Figure 6.
Treatment algorithm [40].

While minimal cases of recurrence have been reported with both techniques, the theoretical disadvantages of the arthroscopic Latarjet are costly, have longer operative time, and have increased difficulty in graft positioning [36, 37]. Several studies explain a greater and more complex learning curve for the arthroscopic Latarjet [37].

Patients treated with arthroscopic Latarjet have less pain in the first 2 weeks postoperatively, but at 1 month they are comparable to the pain experienced by those undergoing open Latarjet. The average time has been reported to be longer for the arthroscopic technique compared to the open technique; however, it has not been determined if this is significant. For screw position and bone locking, there is no improvement with arthroscopic Latarjet according to Horner et al. Only 1% in their study was converted from an arthroscopic to an open procedure due to technical difficulties [38]. One study suggests that conversion rates are quite low once the surgeon has performed a sufficient number of arthroscopic Latarjet procedures [39].

For glenohumeral joint instability, to provide optimal treatment, good preoperative imaging is critical, and based on the degree of one loss and patient expectations White et al. recommend a treatment algorithm (**Figure 6**).

In conclusion, both techniques can be used to successfully treat anterior shoulder instability with similarly low rates of complications, recurrence, and need for revision [34, 41].

7. Rehabilitation and return to physical activity

Rehabilitation and time to return to sport after glenohumeral joint stabilization surgery is one of the most important factors to consider. This includes consideration of psychological, physiological readiness and resilience factors; these are highly linked to the ability to return to sport and the prognosis of the surgery [42, 43].

Weekes et al. showed that 51% of patients treated with arthroscopic stabilization had symptoms of depression on postoperative screening, while these improved by 24% postoperatively; patients who experienced signs of depression at 1 year had lower scores on the WOSI test. Tjong identified several psychological factors that prevent patients from returning to sport. These include re-injury, mood, and self-motivation [42, 43]. Most surgeons base their criteria on time, but Junior et al. found that athletes who underwent objective criteria for return to sport were shown to have lower recurrence rates after arthroscopic stabilization than those who used a decision based on time after surgery [44]. Those undergoing the Latarjet procedure should be followed up with periodic radiographs. Most surgeons obtain radiographs at the first postoperative visit to ensure proper positioning of the graft and fixation device, and at 3 months to evaluate graft union before allowing the patient to undergo specific training [45].

8. Conclusions

As can be seen, different issues are involved in the diagnosis and treatment of anterior shoulder instability. A detailed clinical examination allows us to identify the probable cause of the instability and to select the imaging studies and type of procedure to be performed.

Both arthroscopic and open stabilization techniques are reproducible and have similar recurrence and complication rates. Dynamic stabilization is a useful technique for reducing neurovascular complications. It avoids the decrease in external rotation of the shoulder seen in the Latarjet and allows SLAP type lesions to be managed in the same procedure. However, there are still no studies comparing this technique with the Bankart and Latarjet repair procedures.

Author details

Adrián Aziz Cortés de la Fuente* and Maximiliano Cruz Palacios*
Instituto de Seguridad Social del Estado de México y Municipios (Social Security Institute of the State of Mexico and Municipalities), Toluca, Mexico

*Address all correspondence to: aaziiz_@hotmail.com and max.cruzpalacios@gmail.com

References

[1] Hurley ET, Matache BA, Wong I, Itoi E, Strauss EJ, Delaney RA, et al. Anterior shoulder instability part I-diagnosis, nonoperative management, and Bankart repair-an international consensus statement. Arthroscopy: The Journal of Arthroscopic & Related Surgery. 2022;**38**(2):214-223.e7. DOI: 10.1016/j.arthro.2021.07.022

[2] Parvaresh KC, Vargas-Vila M, Bomar JD, Pennock AT. Anterior glenohumeral instability in the adolescent athlete. JBJS Reviews. 2020;**8**(2):e0080-e0080. DOI: 10.2106/jbjs.rvw.19.00080

[3] Varacallo M, Musto MA, Mair SD. Anterior shoulder instability. In: StatPearls [Internet]. Treasure Island, FL: StatPearls Publishing; Jan-4 Aug 2023. PMID: 30855822

[4] Rockwood CA, Wirth MA. In: Matsen FA, Cordasco FA, Sperling JW, Lippitt SB, editors. The Shoulder. Akron, OH: Saunders; 2009. Hardback ISBN: 9780323698368. eBook ISBN: 9780323698375

[5] Provencher MT, Bhatia S, Ghodadra NS, Grumet RC, Bach BR Jr, Dewing C, et al. Recurrent shoulder instability: Current concepts for evaluation and management of glenoid bone loss. The Journal of Bone and Joint Surgery. 2010;**2**:133-151

[6] Bakhsh W, Nicandri G. Anatomy and physical examination of the shoulder. Sports Medicine and Arthroscopy Review. 2018;**26**(3):e10-e22. DOI: 10.1097/jsa.0000000000000202

[7] Streubel P, Krych A, Simone J, Dahm D, Sperling J, Steinmann S, et al. Anterior glenohumeral instability. Journal of the American Academy of Orthopaedic Surgeons. 2014;**22**(5):283-294

[8] Sheean AJ, De Beer JF, Di Giacomo G, Itoi E, Burkhart SS. Shoulder instability: State of the Art. Journal of ISAKOS [Internet]. 2016 [cited 20 May 2020];**1**(6):347-357. Available from: https://jisakos.bmj.com/content/1/6/347

[9] Parvaresh C, Vargas-Vila K, Bomar JD, Pennock AT. Anterior glenohumeral instability in the adolescent athlete. Journal of Bone and Joint Surgery. 2020;**8**(2):1-10

[10] Di Giacomo G, de Gasperis N, Scarso P. Bipolar bone defect in the shoulder anterior dislocation. Knee Surgery, Sports Traumatology, Arthroscopy. 2015;**24**(2):479-488

[11] Werthel J, Sabatier V, Schoch B, Amsallem L, Nourissat G, Valenti P, et al. Outcomes of the Latarjet procedure for the treatment of chronic anterior shoulder instability: Patients with prior arthroscopic Bankart repair versus primary cases. The American Journal of Sports Medicine. 2019;**48**(1):27-32

[12] Martínez-Montiel O, Valencia-Martínez G, Jasso-Ramírez LA. Reconstrucción con bloque óseo tricortical cadavérico en luxación glenohumeral anterior recurrente con pérdida ósea glenoidea: técnica modificada de Eden Hybinette [Reconstruction with cadaveric tricortical bone block in recurrent anterior glenohumeral dislocation with glenoid bone loss: Modified Eden Hybinette technique]. Acta ortopédica mexicana. 2020;**34**(2):119-122

[13] Cortes-De la Fuente AA, Valencia-Martínez G, Martínez-Montiel O. Treatment results of a modified Eden-Hybinette technique for anterior shoulder instability. Resultados del

tratamiento de una técnica modificada de Eden-Hybinette para la inestabilidad del hombro anterior. Acta ortopédica mexicana. 2021;**35**(6):534-538

[14] Rashid MS, Arner JW, Millett PJ, Sugaya H, Emery R. The Bankart repair: past, present, and future. Journal of Shoulder and Elbow Surgery. 2020;**29**(12):e491-e498. DOI: 10.1016/j.jse.2020.06.012

[15] Bliven K, Parr G. Outcomes of the Latarjet procedure compared with Bankart repair for recurrent traumatic anterior shoulder instability. Journal of Athletic Training. 2018;**53**(2):181-183

[16] Shaha J, Cook J, Song D, Rowles D, Bottoni C, Shaha S, et al. Redefining "critical" bone loss in shoulder instability. The American Journal of Sports Medicine. 2015;**43**(7):1719-1725

[17] Di Giacomo G, Itoi E, S. Burkhart S. Evolving concept of bipolar bone loss and the Hill-Sachs Lesion: From "engaging/non-engaging" lesion to "on-track/off-track" lesion. Art. 2014;**30**(1):90-98

[18] Provencher M, Frank R, Golijanin P, Gross D, Cole B, Verma N et al. Distal tibia allograft glenoid reconstruction in recurrent anterior shoulder instability: Clinical and radiographic outcomes. 2017;**33**:891-897

[19] Burkhart SS, De Beer JF. Traumatic glenohumeral bone defects and their relationship to failure of arthroscopic Bankart repairs: significance of the inverted-pear glenoid and the humeral engaging Hill-Sachs lesion. Arthroscopy: The Journal of Arthroscopic & Related Surgery. 2000;**16**(7):677-694. DOI: 10.1053/jars.2000.17715

[20] Waterman B, Chandler P, Teague E, Provencher M, Tokish J, Pallis M. Short-term outcomes of glenoid bone block augmentation for complex anterior shoulder instability in a high-risk population. 2016;**32**:1784-1790

[21] Galvin JW, Zimmer ZR, Prete AM, Warner JJP. The open Eden-Hybinette procedure for recurrent anterior shoulder instability with glenoid bone loss. Operative Techniques in Sports Medicine. 2019;**27**:95-101. DOI: 10.1053/j.otsm.2019.03.008

[22] Burkhart S, De Beer J, Barth J, Criswell T, Roberts C, Richards D. Results of modified Latarjet reconstruction in patients with anteroinferior instability and significant bone loss. Arthroscopy: The Journal of Arthroscopic & Related Surgery. 2007;**23**(10):1033-1041

[23] Haroun HK, Sobhy MH, Abdelrahman AA. Arthroscopic Bankart repair with remplissage versus Latarjet procedure for management of engaging Hill-Sachs lesions with subcritical glenoid bone loss in traumatic anterior shoulder instability: a systematic review and meta-analysis. Journal of Shoulder and Elbow Surgery. 2020;**29**(10):2163-2174. DOI: 10.1016/j.jse.2020.04.032

[24] Milenin O, Toussaint B. Labral repair augmentation by labroplasty and simultaneous trans-subscapular transposition of the long head of the biceps. Arthroscopy Techniques. 2019;**8**(5):e507-e512. DOI: 10.1016/j.eats.2019.01.010

[25] Collin P, Lädermann A. Dynamic anterior stabilization using the long head of the biceps for anteroinferior glenohumeral instability. Arthroscopy Techniques. 2017;**7**(1):e39-e44. DOI: 10.1016/j.eats.2017.08.049

[26] Collin P, Nabergoj M, Denard PJ, Wang S, Bothorel H, Lädermann A. Arthroscopic biceps transfer to the

glenoid with Bankart repair grants satisfactory 2-year results for recurrent anteroinferior glenohumeral instability in subcritical bone loss. Arthroscopy. 2022;**38**(6):1766-1771. DOI: 10.1016/j.arthro.2021.11.043

[27] de Campos AC, Ângelo AC. All-suture anchor dynamic anterior stabilization produced successful healing of the biceps tendon: A report of 3 cases. JBJS Case Connect. 2021;**11**(1):1-9. DOI: 10.2106/JBJS.CC.20.00149

[28] de Campos AC, Ângelo AC. Onlay dynamic anterior stabilization with biceps transfer for the treatment of anterior glenohumeral instability produces good clinical outcomes and successful healing at a minimum 1 year of follow-up. Arthroscopy, Sports Medicine, and Rehabilitation. 2023;**5**(2):e445-e457. DOI: 10.1016/j.asmr.2023.01.012

[29] Mehl J, Otto A, Imhoff FB, Murphy M, Dyrna F, Obopilwe E, et al. Dynamic anterior shoulder stabilization with the long head of the biceps tendon: A biomechanical study. The American Journal of Sports Medicine. 2019;**47**(6):1441-1450. DOI: 10.1177/0363546519833990

[30] Bokshan SL, Gil JA, DeFroda SF, Badida R, Crisco JJ, Owens BD. Biomechanical comparison of the long head of the biceps tendon versus conjoint tendon transfer in a bone loss shoulder instability model. Orthopaedic Journal of Sports Medicine. 2019;**7**(11):2325967119883549. DOI: 10.1177/2325967119883549

[31] Bottoni CR, Johnson JD, Zhou L, Raybin SG, Shaha JS, Cruz CA, et al. Arthroscopic versus open anterior shoulder stabilization: A prospective randomized clinical trial with 15-year follow-up with an assessment of the glenoid being "on-track" and "Off-Track" as a predictor of failure. The American Journal of Sports Medicine. 2021;**49**(8):1999-2005. DOI: 10.1177/03635465211018212

[32] Chalmers PN, Mascarenhas R, Leroux T, Sayegh ET, Verma NN, Cole BJ, et al. Do arthroscopic and open stabilization techniques restore equivalent stability to the shoulder in the setting of anterior glenohumeral instability? a systematic review of overlapping meta-analyses. Arthroscopy: The Journal of Arthroscopic & Related Surgery. 2015;**31**(2):355-363. DOI: 10.1016/j.arthro.2014.07.00

[33] Bottoni CR, Smith EL, Berkowitz MJ, Towle RB, Moore JH. Arthroscopic versus open shoulder stabilization for recurrent anterior instability: a prospective randomized clinical trial. The American Journal of Sports Medicine. 2006;**34**(11):1730-1737. DOI: 10.1177/0363546506288239

[34] Horner NS, Moroz PA, Bhullar R, Habib A, Simunovic N, Wong I, et al. Open versus arthroscopic Latarjet procedures for the treatment of shoulder instability: a systematic review of comparative studies. BMC Musculoskeletal Disorders. 2018;**19**(1):255. DOI: 10.1186/s12891-018-2188-2

[35] Lafosse L, Boyle S. Arthroscopic Latarjet procedure. Journal of Shoulder and Elbow Surgery. 2010;**19**(2 Suppl):2-12. DOI: 10.1016/j.jse.2009.12.010

[36] Randelli P, Fossati C, Stoppani C, Evola FR, De Girolamo L. Open Latarjet versus arthroscopic Latarjet: clinical results and cost analysis. Knee Surgery, Sports Traumatology, Arthroscopy. 2016;**24**(2):526-532. DOI: 10.1007/s00167-015-3978-9

[37] Cunningham G, Benchouk S, Kherad O, Lädermann A. Comparison of arthroscopic and open Latarjet with a learning curve analysis. Knee Surgery, Sports Traumatology, Arthroscopy. 2016;**24**(2):540-545. DOI: 10.1007/s00167-015-3910-3

[38] Skupiński J, Piechota M, Wawrzynek W, Maczuch J, Babińska A. The Bony Bankart lesion: How to measure the glenoid bone loss. Polish Journal of Radiology. 2017;**82**:58-63

[39] Castricini R, De Benedetto M, Orlando N, Rocchi M, Zini R, Pirani P. Arthroscopic Latarjet procedure: analysis of the learning curve. Musculoskeletal Surgery. 2013;**97**(Suppl 1):93-98. DOI: 10.1007/s12306-013-0262-3

[40] White AE, Patel NK, Hadley CJ, Dodson CC. An algorithmic approach to the management of shoulder instability. JAAOS Global Research & Reviews. 2019;**3**(12):e19.00168. DOI: 10.5435/JAAOSGlobal-D-19-00168

[41] Hurley ET, Lim Fat D, Farrington SK, Mullett H. Open Versus Arthroscopic Latarjet Procedure for Anterior Shoulder Instability: A Systematic Review and Meta-analysis. The American Journal of Sports Medicine. 2019;**47**(5):1248-1253. DOI: 10.1177/0363546518759540

[42] Tjong VK, Devitt BM, Murnaghan ML, Ogilvie-Harris DJ, Theodoropoulos JS. A Qualitative Investigation of Return to Sport After Arthroscopic Bankart Repair: Beyond Stability. The American Journal of Sports Medicine. 2015;**43**(8):2005-2011. DOI: 10.1177/0363546515590222

[43] Weekes DG, Campbell RE, Shi WJ, Giunta N, Freedman KB, Pepe MD, et al. Prevalence of clinical depression among patients after shoulder stabilization: A prospective study. Journal of Bone and Joint Surgery. 2019;**101**(18):1628-1635. DOI: 10.2106/JBJS.18.01460

[44] Drummond Junior M, Popchak A, Wilson K, Kane G, Lin A. Criteria-based return-to-sport testing is associated with lower recurrence rates following arthroscopic Bankart repair. Journal of Shoulder and Elbow Surgery. 2021;**30**(7S):S14-S20. DOI: 10.1016/j.jse.2021.03.141

[45] Matache BA, Hurley ET, Wong I, Itoi E, Strauss EJ, Delaney RA, et al. Anterior shoulder instability part III-revision surgery, rehabilitation and return to play, and clinical follow-up-an international consensus statement. Arthroscopy: The Journal of Arthroscopic & Related Surgery. 2022;**38**(2):234-242.e6. DOI: 10.1016/j.arthro.2021.07.019

Chapter 2

Glenoid Bone Defect in Anterior Shoulder Instability

Svetoslav Dobrilov

Abstract

Bipolar bone defect in shoulder instability are main reason for poor results after arthroscopic stabilization for acute or chronic shoulder instability. Precise quantification of those defects and their interaction to each other should be done, when facing patient with multiple shoulder dislocations. Subsequently treatment should be addressed to clinical and imaging findings. CT and MRI are now "gold standards" for decision making regarding bone defects after multiple shoulder dislocations. Bone transfers are established as reliable surgical option for such patients. They provide opportunity to compensate even large bone defects. Laterjet coracoid transfer is one of the best surgical options with easy technique and reliable results.

Keywords: glenoid bone defect, instability, reconstruction, Laterjet, shoulder dislocation

1. Introduction

Increasing physical activity, especially among young people is reason for respectively, the increase of sport injuries. Shoulder joint, as most mobile joint, is one of the most traumatized joint during sports activities. Shoulder dislocation and shoulder instability are common disorders, that are interrupting normal everyday activities, especially in young athlethes.

Bone defects after shoulder dislocation and recurrent instability are fundamental for diagnostics and treatment of anterior shoulder instability. Precise diagnosis and surgical options are result of proper imaging modalities and the ability of the surgeon to use them. Anterior shoulder dislocation as the reason for shoulder instability affects 40 per 100,000 in men and 15 per 100,000 in women [1]. Results of conservative treatment can lead up to 50% reccurensy [2]. First time dislocators can sustain fracture of anterior glenoid rim or erosion up to 30% of cases [3]. In reccurensy cases described pathologies are increasing up to 86% [4]. Bone defects of anterior glenoid rim (Bankart) and humeral head (Hill-Sachs) are defined as main risk factor for failure of conservative/arthroscopic soft tissue stabilization procedures [5, 6].

Instability of the glenohumeral joint is defined as inability of the humeral head to stay centered into glenoid fossa. This is excessive mobility of joint surfaces to each other, resulting in partial or total dislocation. The difference in partial dislocation is, that articular surfaces still have some contact between and when causative factor is removed, it reduces spontaneous.

In dislocation, translation of the humeral head is so big, that it does not interact with glenoid fossa, respectively it cannot reduce spontaneously.

Definition of shoulder instability comes with proper classification in order to provide proper treatment algorithm. In past decades there are many classifications which are trying to fulfill all requirements – being precise, complete and easy to apply in everyday practice. The closest one, according to literature and our experience, is FEDS classification- it is based on the most important parameters of instability [7] (**Table 1**).

Direction	Ethiology	Severity	Frequency	Pathoanatomy**
Anterior	Traumatic	Pain*	Single episode	Capsule
Posterior	Requires reduction	Subluxation	2–5 episodes	Labrum
Inferior	No reduction requriment	Dsilocation	>5 episodes	Bone
	Atraumatic Positional INvoluntary Habitual Microtraumatic*	Incarcerated	Incarcerated	

**In "overhead" atlethes.*
***Only image detectable.*

Table 1.
Modified FEDS system.

2. Bone defects in anterior shoulder instability

2.1 Pathomorphology of bone loss in anterior shoulder instability

Understanding shoulder instability and its treatment is impossible without knowledge of the pathomorphological changes occurring in shoulder dislocation. The evolution of the latter into shoulder instability depends on many factors acting synchronously. Changes in the anatomical structures responsible for joint stability are directly related to the specific anatomy of the shoulder joint.

Main topic of this chapter is glenoid bone defect and because of that, soft tissue pathology will not be discussed.

Bone deficiency after sigle or multiple shoulder dislocations is considered to be important factor for reccurensy of instability after soft-tissue stabilization procedures [8, 9]. Thus, it has to be diagnosed and evaluated before any treatment. Multiple studies have reported reccurensy of instability due to glenoid bone defect ranging from 36% to 93.7%, with the rate directly proportional to the number of episodes of instability [10]. Patients with "minimal" glenoid loss (up to 13%) have reported poor functional outcomes after primary soft-tissue stabilization [11]. Similar data have been reported in Hill-Sachs defect, reaching even to 100%, in combine bone defects. Because of that, bone morphology and integrity are very important factors influencing outcomes after surgical treatment of shoulder instability [12].

The amount of bone loss and the recurrence rate often after soft tissue stabilization account for the preference for bony reconstructions in patients with significant bone loss [13, 14]. The frequency of bone defects varies according to literature data, depending on the evaluation methodology used. In patients with anterior instability, the frequency of glenoid bone loss is between 49 and 86%, and of humeral defects - even up to 100% [15].

Bipolar bone defects are almost obligatory finding in patients with anterior glenohumeral instability [13, 14]. They lead to instability because, altering the congruence of the glenohumeral joint and the function of the static stabilizers, like glenoid surface, congruence, etc. In physically active patients, their frequency is particularly high, because of the increased activity, age and potential for injuries of the respective discipline. Contact sports (rugby, martial arts, wrestling, bars, etc.) and overhead sports (basketball, volleyball, handball, etc.) can lead to high-energy traumatic dislocations and are usually accompanied by significant bone defects [16]. In contrast, the rate of bone loss is much less in non-contact sports (track and field), where chondrolabral and pure labral injuries predominate. Other situations associated with significant glenoid bone loss are post-convulsive conditions and bike/motorcycle trauma [17].

Glenoid bone loss is among the causes of glenohumeral instability and one of the most important factors responsible for failure and recurrence after arthroscopic stabilization [12]. A high percentage of patients with chronic anterior glenohumeral instability have some type of glenoid bone loss. Recognizing bone loss and determining its degree is of great importance, with planning individualized treatment algorithm. Detecting chronic bone loss is important for several reasons. Unlike an acute Bankart lesion, a chronic one may be associated with erosive glenoid wear and chronic medialization of the anterior-inferior capsuloligamentous complex. Humeral bone defects also multuply frequency of instability [15].

Patients with more than three dislocations or with persistence of more than 4 hours in a dislocated state are suspected of significant posttraumatic bone loss [16]. A history of frequent recurrent dislocations, especially during daily activities, is suspicious for a bony defect. It is recommended, that bone loss be differentiated as acute or chronic. This is done with a careful history and X-ray examination. Although acute large bony Bankart lesions cause clinically significant bone loss, they can be treated successfully with open or arthroscopic techniques of internal fixation. Bigliani et al. reported good results after anatomic repositioning and fixation of glenoid rim fragments in accute setting. Thus, the resistance of the glenoid against axial load and, respectively, the arch of movement is restored. Missing that moment, bone loss is tramsfering from acute to chronic and the function of the shoulder is reversibly affected by significant bone loss.

Bony defects of the anterior glenoid are creating mismatch between the articular surfaces, leading to increased anterior translation of the humeral head with minimal force [5]. The difference in the length of the articular surfaces has a negative effect on the ability of the glenoid to resist axial loading. Bone deficiency also decreases the concavity of the glenoid fossa, increasing the inability to hold the humeral head in translation [5]. In the presence of bipolar bone defects, the instability is further aggravated.

In 1998, Bigliani et al. [17] were the first to introduce the term bony Bankart when defining an anteroinferior bony fragment of the glenoid with a preserved insertion of the inferior glenohumeral ligament (Biliani type I). Biliani type II is a fragment with poor consolidation and firm connection to the ligamentous complex. The third type of defect is the erosive one with two subtypes: III A - with defect size below 25% and III B - above 25% of the total glenoid surface.

Radiologically, chronic unstable glenohumeral joints, have about 90% bone loss [18]. Based on arthroscopic and CT findings, Sugaya et al. found that, only

10% have intact glenohumeral joints, 40% have erosive-compression defects of the glenoid and 50% - with bony- Bankart [14]. Itoi et al. stated that a lesion of 21% of the glenoid length is reducing the stability provided by the glenoid by 50%, corresponding to an 18% deficit on West Point radiographic projection and a 50% loss of glenoid depth determined by CT [19]. In a cadaver study, autors defined that the position of the defect was usually at 4:30 o'clock (in right joints) and was more anterior than anteroinferior [20]. Bone defects greater than 21% of the glenoid width significantly reduce stability, compromise Bankart reconstruction, and therefore are indicated for bone augmentation [21]. The localization of this "critical" defect is predominantly anterior rather than anteroinferior [20]. More recent studies have shown a significant decrease in stability after defect formation beyond 26% of the glenoid width (20% of the length) [21]. In addition, stability after soft tissue reconstruction (Bankart) is significantly reduced in the presence of such a defect (**Figure 1**) [21].

Bony defects between 0 and 15% of the glenoid width (< 3–4 mm) are usually imperceptible to regular patients (excluding high-level athletes), while defects greater than 20% (>6-10 mm) are clinically significant.

The concept of the "inverted pear" proposed by Burkhart [5] provides an explanation of what is clinically significant bone loss. This is when a large bony Bankart lesion turns the normal shape of the glenoid (pear-shaped, with a larger transverse dimension at its bottom) into a so-called "inverted pear" (**Figure 1**). This form is recognizable either arthroscopically or with imaging studies (CT, MRI).

The geometric center of the inferior glenoid it is defined as "bearing point" and this is the anatomical landmark for accurate arthroscopic determination of the radius of the glenoid. This is done through an anterior superior-lateral arthroscopic portal, with the introduction of a calibrated probe through the posterior portal. Burkhart and De Beer [5] used the "bearing point" as a reference point for arthroscopic measurement of glenoid loss. Sugaya et al. [14] demonstrated that the inferior part of the glenoid is almost circular in shape (about 24 mm in diameter) and determined the size of the defect along the missing portion of this circle. These two methods determine the degree of bone loss without information about the native shape of the glenoid in question.

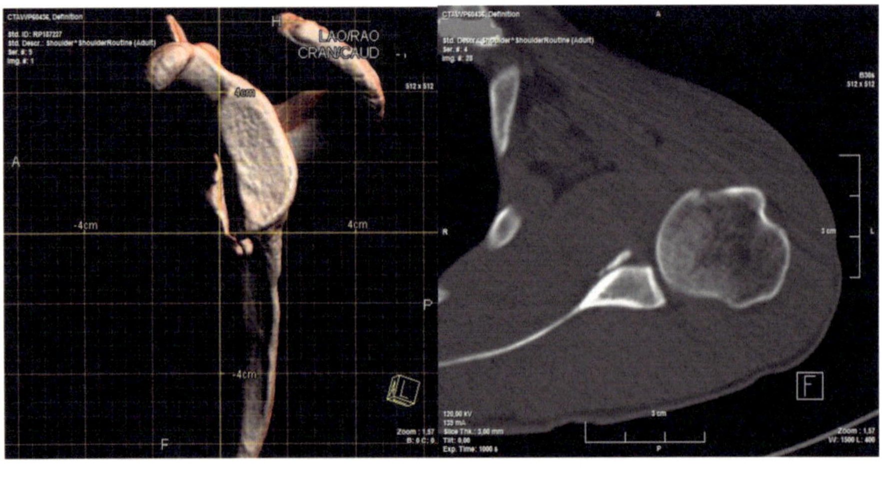

Figure 1.
Typical location of the glenoid defect in anterior shoulder instability and creating " inverted pear" glenoid.

Anatomical studies of the glenoid are extensive, with two of them referring to its inferior part [22]. De Wilde et al. confirm again the round shape of this part of the glenoid, the center of which is Asaki's tubercle - the underlying bone of the so-called "bearing point"/"bare spot" [23].

Aigner et al. [24] measured the distances from this point to the cartilaginous edge of the glenoid and found that most of the "bearing spots" were eccentrically located and therefore not a reliable guide in determining the amount of bone loss. Conversely, Burkhart et al. [5] define precisely the "bare spot" for the geometric center of the inferior glenoid. The measurements of Aigner et al. differ in millimeters, which makes the differences negligible and confirms the reliability of the concept of the "bare spot". Huysmans et al. explain the differences in the lengths of the distance from the center to the glenoid rim with the triangular shape of the labrum and the uneven density of the underlying bone. Therefore, when the distance from the "bare spot" to the posterior labrum, in patients with a detached anterior labrum, is equal to the distance from the "bare spot" to the anterior glenoid rim, a small bone defect is already present [25]. It is for this reason that the concept of the "bare spot" can be used to determine the degree of glenoid loss, especially in combination with CT or MRI.

When discussing bone deficiency in anterior shoulder instability it is obligatory to include defects of the humeral head, because both defects interact dynamically in shoulder motion. Thus, when treating glenoid deficiency, we need to consider humeral head defects either.

The Hill-Sachs lesion is an impression fracture of the posterosuperior, lateral part of the humeral head, first described by Malgen in 1855 and studied radiographically in detail by Hill and Sachs in 1940. It can occur with any dislocation because the impaction of the soft humeral head on the hard bone of the glenoid (**Figure 2**).

The frequency of the defect is between 65% and 67% after a primary dislocation and 84–93% after a recurrent one. This frequency is actually highly dependent on radiographic projections. On anteroposterior views, it is reported in only 7% of primary dislocations, but on MRI it is 93% [26]. The frequency of lesions in young patients with traumatic dislocations in several arthroscopic series ranges between 47% and 100% [14]. Hill-Sachs defects are graded depending on the percentage of involvement of the humeral head: less than 20% (small defects); between 20% and 45% (medium) and above 45% (major defects). The critical threshold of the humeral

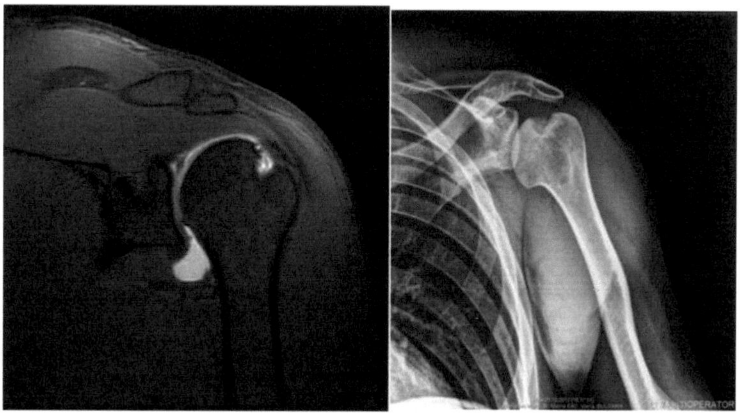

Figure 2.
Hill-Sachs defect.

defect is still a subject of debate - 4 cm in length, 20–25% of the surface of the humeral head and about 250–1000 mm3 volume of the defect [27].

According to Saito, the defect is located between 0 mm and 24 mm from the tip of the humeral head. Spatschil presents a relationship between the number of dislocations and the frequency of defects. In patients with only one dislocation, the incidence of Hill-Sachs defects is around 67%, whereas in patients with more than one dislocation, the incidence increase up to 84% [4]. That's why there is direct proportional dependence between the number of dislocations and the size of the defect.

Accurate assessment of the size of the Hill-Sachs lesion and its interaction with glenoid bone loss improved with Itoi's introduction of the glenoid track concept [21]. Itoi [28] was the first to determine the "critical size" of the glenoid biomechanically in cadavers. With a fixed scapula, movement of the humeral head relative to the glenoid is reproduced in a position of elevation from 0° to 60°, which corresponds to a position of 90° to the body and maximum external rotation. "Glenoid track" represents the contact area between the humeral head and the glenoid fossa in the various phases of motion—the varying degrees of elevation at maximum external rotation and maximum extension. This end position is critical for instability due to tension on the capsuloligamentous complex and prevention against anterior translation of the humeral head. It is in this position that patients feel a positive apprehension test. During the movement from inferomedial to superolateral, an "imprint" is formed on the humeral head from the glenoid fossa - the so-called "glenoid track". As long as the Hill-Sachs defect is located within the limits of glenoid track, there is no risk that the anterior edge of the glenoid will "engage" the defect and result in a lever mechanism, resp. dislocation. It is classified as an "on track" lesion. However, if the above mentioned defect exceeds the size of glenoid track, there is a risk of "engagement" with the anterior edge of the glenoid and resulting in instability. This type of pathology is classified as an "off track" lesion.

The distance from the medial edge of the contact zone to the medial edge of the rotator cuff is approximately 18 mm, or 84% of the glenoid width at 60° abduction [21].

Itoi et al. [29] measured glenoid track also in vivo by MRI. The position of the hand was put in seven different degrees of elevation with maximal external rotation of the limb maintained. Computer analysis showed that localization of the medial edge of the glenoid track was 93%, 85%, 82%, and 82% at 60°, 90°, 120°, and 150° elevation, respectively. Values at 90° elevation are closest to those measured on cadavers. Burkhart and De Beer's [5] concept of an engaging/non-engaging defect is fully consistent with Itoi's [21] concept of the "glenoid track". Together, both concepts explain and evaluate the interaction of bipolar bone defects on dynamic shoulder function. Because ot that, these two concepts are "milestones" of understanding bone deficiency in shoulder instability.

Assessment of bone loss by 3D CT is an essential tool when evaluating patient with instability. There are numerous biomechanical studies on the mechanisms of bipolar bone defects. However, there is a lack of data demonstrating the pathomorphological evolution of these defects in a specific patient.

Nakagawa performed such a study on 204 shoulders evaluated by CT preoperatively, postoperatively, and postrecurrence. The size of the defect is undoubtedly a determinant, but the development of these defects over time also has therapeutic importance for predicting instability. The author reported a mean glenoid defect value of 2.2% with a fragmentary type of bone loss in half of the cases. The high frequency of Hill-Sachs defect (66% of cases) against such a small glenoid defect is cofusing. The overall incidence of bipolar bone loss is approximately 30%. This is somewhat at odds with other studies, that postulate a predominantly glenoid defect and much less Hill-Sachs lesions. Regarding the influence of the degree of dislocation/subluxation, Nakagawa reported a significant difference in the presence and size of Hill-Sachs lesions in dislocated and subluxated joints. This is not absolute for glenoid bone loss. CT findings after a first episode of instability show a logical 100% increase in the amount of bone loss measured (in the study from 0–10% to 6–17%). Regarding the occurrence of Hill-Sachs lesions, no significant difference was found, although the size of the loss increased.

Multiple studies based on 3D CT have shown a directly proportional relationship between the size of bipolar bone defects, age, and the number of dislocations [30]. The frequency of occurrence of these defects increases with increasing episodes of instability. Nakagawa studied bipolar bone loss in 153 shoulders and reported a population prevalence of over 56%. Including the isolated defects, the total frequency of bone defects becomes more than 85%. On average, the presence of bipolar bone loss in patients with a primary episode of instability is 34%, while in a recurrent episode it is already 62% and increases proportionally with the number of episodes [30].

The question arises as to the timing of the stabilization procedure. Is such an intervention necessary immediately after the first dislocation, when the defect is CT evaluated, or to wait for the first epizode of recurrence and the formation of already "critical" bone loss, preventing further enlargement of the defect and increasing the risk of instability after already done stabilization. Large Hill-Sachs defects are also more common after instability recurrence. Nakagawa reported that 12% of male professional athletes with recurrent instability had off-track Hill-Sachs [31]. This suggests that these defects develop from several episodes of instability, rather than a single one.

When we define glenoid bone loss as "fragmentary" or "erosive" type, it should be kept in mind that very often small bone fragments undergo resorption and thus loss after recurrence is defined as "erosive" type. In Nakagawa's studies, a bone fragment was not always differentiated in the first dislocation, and the anterior glenoid rim often showed signs of a compression fracture without a bone fragment present [32]. This is may be because of the different timing in appearance of the patient. That's why it is very important, patients with shoulder dislocations to be closely followed-up and evaluated for glenoid deficiency.

Randelli [33] did an extensive analysis of risk factors for instability, particularly after arthroscopic soft-tissue stabilization. The age of the patient is the most common reason for recurrence. Many autors reported a significant negative correlation between postoperative instability and age at first operation: 25% in patients younger than 20 years; 20% at 20 years - 30 years; 7% in patients between 30 and 40 years. Taking the 20th year as borderline, the frequency of recurrence below this age is 33.6%, while above it - 11.8%. Porcellini [34] reported a 10% risk of recurrence in males, compared to 2.8% in females. The overall recurrence rate in men is about 15%, and in women 8.7%. The number of dislocations is also an important prognostic marker for the risk of recurrence. According to Imhoff [35] the risk is directly proportional to the number of preoperative dislocations, reaching a 44% with more than 10 dislocations. Other series give similar data at baseline of 5 dislocations [36]. There is no significant relationship between the type and number of anchors used in arthroscopic stabilization and the risk of recurrence [37].

2.2 Imaging and quantification of glenoid defects

Accurate identification and quantification of both glenoid bone loss and the presence of a Hill-Sachs defect is essential in the diagnosis and therapeutic approach of anterior shoulder instability, as it is directly related to functional treatment outcomes. The ability to correctly diagnose and treat these potential bony defects of the glenohumeral joint is based on multiple factors—the patient's history, physical findings, and the various imaging modalities in a clinical setting that are fundamental to a successful outcome. There are multiple methods for quantifying bone loss based on imaging or arthroscopy, and anyone involved in this pathology should consider all bone loss imaging options, their specificity, and sensitivity.

Standard radiographs are the initial imaging of the patient with shoulder instability. While some studies recommend standard radiographs, diagnostic sensitivity, specificity, and accuracy can be greatly influenced by patient positioning during the examination.

In studies reporting the accuracy and reliability of specific radiographic projections, the axillary view, West Point View, true AP view, and Bernageau projection are those that would be useful. Of these, the Bernageau view is reported to be the most accurate and reliable when compared with 3D CT images (**Figure 3**) [19, 38]. A disadvantage is the ignorance of the projection itself by the X-ray laboratory technicians and the poor imaging of the lower bony lesions of the glenoid face [13]. Edwards et al. [13] propose a classification of glenoid loss in this projection into 3 groups: fracture, "cliff" and "blunt angle", but they do not determine its size. Bernageau view represents radiographic projection of the glenoid, which is compared to the healthy contralateral side and serves to calculate glenoid bone loss. This technique is easy to apply and has a sensitivity and specificity of over 90% [13]. With the developing of 3D-CT and MRI, the calculation of bone loss has become more accurate, and many authors have proposed protocols for its determination [39]. Due to popularity of CT imageing, Bernageau view it is not standard procedure, but it should be kept in concideration.

In general, standard radiographs are unreliable relative to modalities such as 3D CT in quantifying glenoid deficiency, which may affect the therapeutic algorithm. Therefore, it is not recommended that, standard radiographs to be used as the sole method for diagnosing glenoid bone loss.

Several methodologies exist in the literature to quantify the extent of glenoid bone loss. These techniques are based on surface area measurements or based on glenoid diameter. The general concept of measuring glenoid bone loss is the understanding

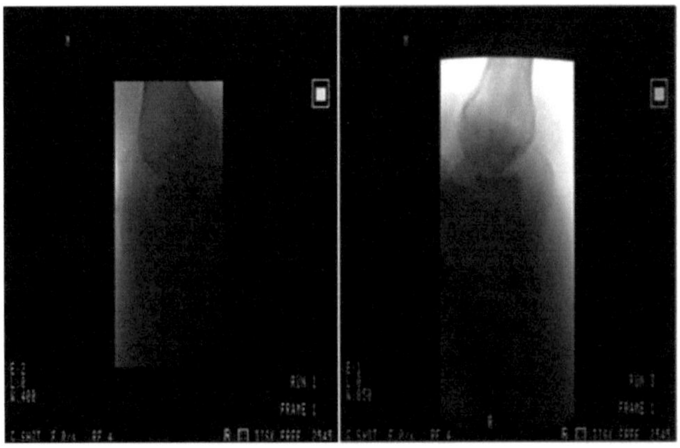

Figure 3.
Bernageau view. Uninjured side (left) and unstable side (wright).

that, the inferior glenoid in the "en face" view resembles a true circle and that the degree of bone loss can be calculated using the geometric properties of a circle or by comparing the ratio of measurements in the healthy, contralateral shoulder [40]. Although there is a lack of consensus and heterogeneity in the literature on the method of measurement, seventeen different methods are available in practice [41].

All methods calculate the ratio of glenoid surface and missing bone on 2D images. Thirteen methods were based on unilateral glenoid measurement and four were based on bilateral measurement. Sixteen methods performed measurements using the glenoid surface (sagittal "en face" view of the glenoid) and one method used the glenoid rim (sagittal view). Eleven of the methods used a reference distance that was divided, 5 methods calculated the defect that was divided by a reference surface, and 1 method used the position of the defect to quantify glenoid bone loss [41].

All methodologies have similar characteristics focused over the glenoid surface in "en face "view. One of the most popular and reliable method is the "ideal circle" (**Figure 4**).

Other reproducible technique is "diameter" method (**Figure 5**).

2.2.1 Surface-based methods

The amount of bone loss of the glenoid face is estimated by surface area methodology using so called "ideal" circle, which is not covered by best-fitting circle Sugaya

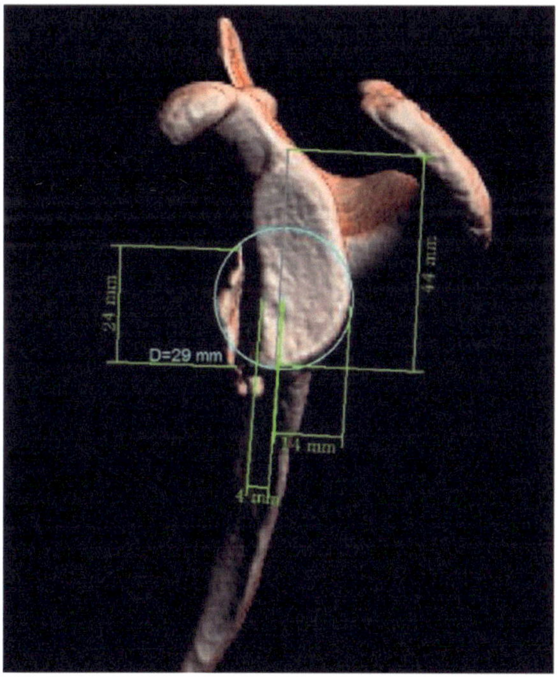

Figure 4.
Method of the "ideal" circle - bare spot method, one-sided. On a sagittal projection, the longitudinal axis from the supraglenoid tubercle to the inferior glenoid rim is determined. It is drawn perpendicularly through the widest part of the inferior glenoid. The intersection of the two lines is the so-called "bare spot" and it is the center of a circle. Bone loss was defined as the ratio of anterior (AD) to posterior distance (PD) using the formula [(PD-AD)/(2xPD)] x 100 [41].

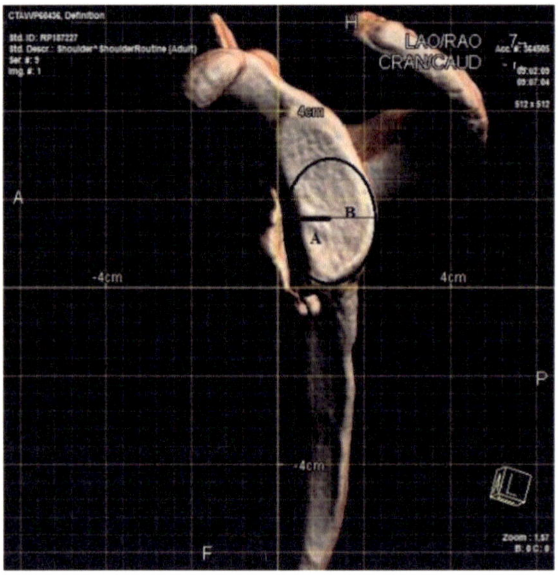

Figure 5.
Method of the "ideal" circle (diameter method), one-sided. On a sagittal projection, the transverse axis of the glenoid is drawn and a circle is placed that most accurately fits between 3' and 9' o'clock of the inferior glenoid. A line perpendicular to the transverse axis is drawn until it reaches the bone defect (A). The diameter of the circle (B) is also determined. Bone loss is calculated using the formula (B-A/B) x 100 [41].

et al. promote a "circle method" for determining bone loss, which was calculated by dividing the area not filled by the glenoid by the surface area of the best-fit circle [40]. Baudi upgrade this technique to method known as the PICO: calculation of the area of the glenoid loss by the area of the healthy contralateral surface of the glenoid, defined by two identical best fit circles [42]. The PICO method has been reported to be highly accurate and reliable in assessing bone loss and has also been shown to be clinically more useable than linear techniques when performed on 3D CT images [42, 43]. PICO technique needs bilateral CT, and some studies reported equal result to MRI, considered as more favorable in clinical setting [44]. It should be noted that calculations using the surface method require more sophisticated software and are more complex than linear methods.

Surface-based measurements are considered as reliable and precise in terms of glenoid bone loss.

2.2.2 Diameter (linear-based) techniques

They are convenient, because they do not require sophisticated image processing software and can be used instantly in clinical practice [45]. These methods, even can be used intraoperatively using arthroscopically assisted measurements. Several variants of linearly based models have been described in the literature. Estimation of bone loss can be done using the contralateral arm or using the "ideal" circle method. The first option can be useful, as no major differences between the two arms have been reported in the morphology of the glenoid region. This does not apply to cases with bilateral involvement [25]. In comparison, the "ideal" circle methodology, with an emphasis on absent bone loss of width, is applied only to the pathological shoulder by estimating the width of the glenoid face and overlapping with the "ideal circle" [45].

New studies report significant reliability of the glenoid index (SI/AP) for assessment of glenoid bone loss. This method is based on the ratio of the measured widths of the pathological and healthy glenoid [16]. Some autors did not find statistically significant differences between the calculations with this methodology and the measurement technique based on surface area in patients with bone loss greater than 6%. They noted that, although not significantly, when the rate of bone loss increased, the differences in measurements also increased [45]. The position of the bone defect affects accuracy of quantifying bone loss in linear measurements, due to presentation only in frontal plane. Bone loss in lower glenoid can be underestimated if defect is located oblique to the frontal plane of the glenoid [46].

Diameter-based measurements can overestimate glenoid bone loss [45]. The "perfect" circle technique has been argued to be inaccuracy, due to an incorrect geometric formula, that would more accurately be applied to calculate the area of a square rather than a circle [47].

In some series, these inaccuracies ranged between 15 and 25%. Because of that, unnecessary bone augmentation may occur due to an exaggeration of bone loss that exceeds the critical threshold of 20–21% for recurrent instability [47]. CT imaging is the most extensively studied modality for assessing bone loss in shoulder instability [46]. Although CT has some well known disadvantages as increased ionizing radiation than other modalities, few studies support its replacement [14, 16]. Many studies show superiority of the CT to other modalities. This often "enforces" 3D CT methodology as the "gold" standard [48]. 3D CT has almost perfect specificity in estimating bone loss [14, 49].

3D CT is reported to be a more accurate and reliable modality than two dimension techniques [48]. The "en face" view of the glenoid fossa, provided by 3D, gives more precise estimation, using surface measurement methods. In contrast, 2D CT images are affected by scapular tilt, which alters the "en face" projection of the glenoid and affects the accuracy of the calculations [48].

Any inclination of the en-face view results in a change of the measured surface and the diameter of the "ideal" circle. Although superior, inferior, and posterior scapular tilts tend to reduce the actual defect, anterior tilts have no such relationship, even the opposite. This leads to underestimation in the first case and overestimation of the defect in the second case. Vertical tilt, in particular, has a significant effect even at 5° malrotation. From a clinical point of view, these changes are not always significant. Naturally, changes in defect measurement are directly proportional to scapular inclination [48].

2.2.3 Arthroscopic evaluation

The term "bare spot" as anatomical center of the glenoid was introduced by Burkhart [50]. This is done during shoulder arthroscopy and it relies to the fact that posterior rim of the glenoid face is intact and can be used as a reverence point measuring the center of the glenoid fossa. Using calibrated probe, author has validated the accuracy of the measurement, compared to 3D CT [51, 52].

However, some studies have shown that, this point could be inconsistent and even absent in some patients up to 48% [53]. Other authors noted that, "bare spot" can be eccentrically located, thus leading to overestimation of the glenoid bone loss. Because of that literature does not recommend to use this method as a single tool.

There is controversy in the literature what is the ideal method for assessing the bone deficiency in glenohumeral instability. In a recent systematic review, Walter et al. compared the efficacy of different imaging methods for quantifying glenoid bone loss. A review of 1425 shoulders concluded that CT (2D/3D) and MRI provide accurate measurement of bone loss in shoulder instability. There is no complete consensus regarding the so-called “gold standard” ac its determination [41, 54].

Regarding the best way to quantify glenoid bone loss, consensus of leading experts, stated that “en face” view of the glenoid face using 3D CT provides the most accurate assessment of the glenoid bone defect. Regarding methods for calculation the size of the defect, 86% of the experts concluded that all the different options available, including the surface area method, the superimposed circle method, the PICO method, etc. are sufficiently reliable [12, 41].

2.2.4 ISIS (instability severity index score) total

In a prospective study, Balg and Boileau proposed the ISIS-score as a way to predict outcomes after arthroscopic stabilization of anterior shoulder instability [55]. In a 10-point preoperative scoring system, risk factors leading to an increased risk of recurrence (also after arthroscopic Bankart) are: patient age less than 20 years at the time of surgery; professional or contact sports; hyperlaxity; Hill-Sachs lesion visible on anteroposterior view of the shoulder ac external rotation and/or loss of the sclerotic contour of the inferior glenoid (**Table 2**).

Age	under 20 yrs. – 2 pts	above 20 yrs. – 0 pts
Sport	Professional- 2 pts	Recreative- 0 pts
Type of sport	Martial / over-head - 1 pts.	Other - 0 pts
Laxity	Hyperlaxity –1 pts	Normal –0 pts
HS defect	positive in ER - 2 pts	Negative in ER – 0 pts
Glenoid	Loss of anteroinferior contour - 2 pts.	No loss – 0 pts

Table 2.
ISIS score.

Since the introduction of the ISIS-score as a predictor of recurrence, multiple studies to validate this score have shown inconclusive data and a lack of consensus. A total ISIS score of less than 4 points is significantly more accurate, than the defined base-limit of 6 points [44, 56].

Dekker performed an extensive review of 217 patients over a 5-year period with arthroscopic stabilization to determine the reliability of the instability severity index score (ISIS) for assessing the risk of recurrent instability. The analysis of patients is based on the main points of the ISIS-score:

1. number of instability episodes,

2. general period of instability,

3. presence and degree of glenoid bone loss,

4. presence and degree of Hill-Sachs defect.

The evaluation systems used in the study are Western Ontario Shoulder Instability Index (WOSI), Single Assessment Numerical Evaluation (SANE) and American Shoulder and Elbow Society scores (ASES). The results of the study indicated no correlation between treatment outcomes and the measured ISIS total. The mean glenoid loss measured in the series was less than 14.5%, which was expected to be lower in patients with good functional outcome, mean Hill-Sachs defect volume greater than 1.3 cm3, and duration of symptoms greater than 3 months. This led the study authors to recommend a revision of the ISIS score, incorporating factors that have increasing weight in deciding on a therapeutic approach. Of particular importance are the degree of glenoid loss and the volume of the Hill-Sachs defect. Loppini did a large controlled 5-year study showing the protective role of a fixed baseline of 3 points, with success rates on this basis of 93.7% [56].

Accurate identification and quantification of both glenoid surface loss and a potential Hill-Sachs lesion is essential in the treatment of anterior shoulder instability, as it directly affects patients outcomes. In a so called first-time dislocator or patient with a history of multiple subluxations, the suspected bony defect should be evaluated comprehensively including soft tissues either.

There are multiple methods for quantifying bone loss, and the surgeon must be aware of both the advantages and disadvantages of each imaging modality when it comes to the accuracy of identifying glenoid bone loss and accurately quantifying the size of bony lesions.

3. Operative treatment for shoulder instability with bone deficiency

Surgical treatment of bone loss in anterior shoulder instability aims to restore the deficit and achieve joint stability. There are several basic operative techniques that can be summarized as: "bone pathology - bone surgery". Once the degree of bone loss has been precisely determined, the method of bone augmentation is a matter of choice for the surgeon, depending on his capabilities and available technical support, as well as the patient's profile.

Treatment of anterior shoulder instability is generally based on two types of operative techniques: anatomic and nonanatomic reconstruction. The anatomical reconstruction aims to restore the glenoid labrum to its anatomical position and achieve optimal tension of the capsulolabral complex. These techniques currently are performed arthroscopically.

Nonanatomic techniques are stabilizing the joint through bone augmentation and increasing the glenoid articular surface, preventing of excessive humeral translation, and stabilization of the joint through isolation of the humeral bone defect. The current understanding of bone loss in shoulder instability, recommends operative techniques to be addressed to the "bipolar bone loss" and not to each one separately. This is because, both bone defects interact dynamically and it would not be appropriate to isolate the treatment for each of the types. This is the reason why this chapter examines the individual operative techniques and their effect on the bone damage of the glenoid-humeral head pair.

3.1 Coracoid transfer: Laterjet

Coracoid transfer - Laterjet was first described in 1958 in the treatment of anterior shoulder instability and involves trasfering the coracoid process over the formed glenoid defect along with its adjacent musculature. The main effects achieved with this technique are:

1. bone replacement of the existing defect and increase of the contact surface of the glenoid with the humeral head. This is how "isolation" of the humeral defect is achieved and its engaging is prevented ("glenoid track concept ");

2. the movement of the coracoid muscles over the lower edge of the subscapularis muscle causes the muscle to "stretch" and thus to stabilize the joint;

3. the so-called "sling effect" - the tendon of the coracoid muscles achieves a "retaining" effect at 90° abduction and 90° external rotation, providing additional stability of the joint by preventing the engaging of the humeral bone defect at this "most unstable" position.

Gradually over time, two main variants of coracoid transfer have been established: open and arthroscopic techniques. Open techniques have been popularized due to consistent postoperative results, relatively less need for surgical expertise, and predictable postoperative complications. The advantages of the arthroscopic technique are less surgical trauma, better visualization and the ability to address concomitant soft tissue injuries. The most common disadvantages are the need for a "learning curve" for the surgeon and more sophisticated technical support.

A number of authors recommend the following treatment algorithm for bipolar bone defects. With glenoid loss ≤13% and the presence of a small "on track" Hill–Sachs, arthroscopic stabilization is recommended. Glenoid loss ≤13% and medium-sized "off track" Hill–Sachs is an indication for arthroscopic stabilization and remplissage. Surgeons experienced in arthroscopy advocate the recommendation for arthroscopic variant of Laterjet transfer. With glenoid loss over 13% and a small "on track" Hill–Sachs – arthroscopic Laterjet technique. The combination of glenoid loss greater than 13% and moderate/large "off track" Hill–Sachs lesions are indications for an open Laterjet technique or free bone graft and replissage [33, 57].

The indications for arthroscopic Laterjet stabilization are:

- Isolated anterior glenoid loss >13%
- Anterior glenoid loss <13% associated with a Bankart lesion
- Anterior glenoid loss >10% and < 20% with an ISIS score of 3–6 points
- First episode of shoulder dislocation no more than 3 years ago
- No more than 5 dislocations

Nonanatomic bone techniques are the subject of extensive debate in the literature. A systematic review of 46 series involving 3211 shoulders showed low rates of recurrence of instability after bone augmentation compared with arthroscopic Bankart [58]. A biomechanical study of the effectiveness of variations of coracoid transfer (Bristow or Laterjet) demonstrated the superiority of Laterjet in restoring stability and reducing the risk of recurrence [59].

The "congruent-arc" modification, which rotates the graft by 90°, has several advantages over the classical one: it restores the radius of curvature of the glenoid face, thus reducing the superior translation of the head and allowing compensation of larger defects. Similar comparisons have been made between the remplisage technique and Laterjet in engaging Hill-Sachs defects.

Ali compared the overall functional outcome after open and arthroscopic Latarjet stabilization by assessing range of motion, strength, and clinical outcomes using the Rowe, WOSI, and visual analog scale (VAS) scoring systems. The author makes an additional assessment radiographically. The most important finding of this study is that both open and arthroscopic techniques produce similar overall functional and radiographic results [60].

In a comparative meta-analysis, Hurley found no significant difference in functional outcomes and complications between arthroscopic and open coracoid transfer (Latarjet) [60]. Data from the systematic review show the same parameters for both techniques: low recurrence and complication rates. Given the greater technical complexity, the arthroscopic version of the Latarjet has been shown to be safe and suitable as an alternative to the open one. It is important to emphasize the significant learning curve for the use of the arthroscopic Laterjet, which suggests its use in large centers with experienced arthroscopists available. With the open technique, the author found a lower frequency of persistent apprehension test, which he explained by the higher frequency of patients returning to sports, especially contact one. Potential benefits of the arthroscopic technique for coracoid transfer lie in less postoperative pain. However, this does not always reflect in less use of analgetics, especially with an opioid component [61, 62].

The financial aspect of the arthroscopic technique continues to be a consideration. Randelli's analysis shows a 3 times higher cost of the arthroscopic versus the open technique, which is an obstacle to the increasing popularity of this technique even in the USA [63]. In both techniques, the accurate positioning of the coracoid process is considered one of the critical steps of the Latarjet technique. Medialized offset of the graft can lead to permanent instability, while lateralization of the graft potentially speed-up degenerative changes,because of increased contact with the humeral head [64, 65]. Optimal graft position is below the glenoid equator, neither too medial nor too lateral, less than 10 mm from the articular cartilage. Visualization of the glenoid for positioning may be more difficult with the open technique, however, many of the technical steps are more easily accomplished with an open exposure. The advantage of the arthroscopic technique is the visualization of the entire glenoid articular surface, which reduces the risk of graft malposition [66].

Graft resorption is one of the most common complications after coracoid transfer and is reported as high as 63.9% in the literature. This consequence has a controversial clinical significance for recurrence of instability and appears to be greater in patients with greater glenoid bone loss and after arthroscopic technique [67]. Conversely, graft resorption in some series is seen more often after open reconstruction compared to arthroscopic. A significant correlation was found between the rate of graft resorption and the positive apprehension test postoperatively, but it did not correlate with the other functional results [68].

3.2 Free tricortical iliac graft

In case of significant glenoid bone loss, one of the preferred stabilization techniques is the open or arthroscopic Eden-Hybinette. This procedure is done with a tricortical iliac graft and has been shown to produce good results, with low rates of recurrent instability. Indications for this technique include severe glenoid loss (> 40%), recurrent instability after Latarjet or distal tibial allotransplantation, patients with abnormal coracoid morphology [69, 70].

Eden-Hybinette offers the possibility of tailoring the size of the bone augment to match the corresponding glenoid bone loss. Furthermore, this technique exculdes the risk of potential allogeneic contamination and is less expensive, despite the obvious disadvantage of donor site morbidity. Arthroscopic reconstruction with a tricortical iliac graft was introduced by Sugaya. Soon after, other authors such as Taverna and Kraus reported excellent short-term results with this technique [71]. Both versions of the Eden-Hybinette technique – arthroscopic or open technique – are equally effective [72].

A study by Malahias on different techniques for processing and fixation of a tricortical iliac graft showed that, regardless of the type of fixation and shaping of the graft, this technique gave excellent functional results and low rates (6%) of reoperation [73]. In addition, all important aspects of shoulder stabilization techniques such as: recurrences (4.8%), positive apprehension test (4.8%), nonunion (2.2%), osteolysis (0.4%), etc. are very low. Based on the meta-analysis, the author recommends the technique as safe and predictable in terms of functional results and complications. Bone augmentation of the glenoid with a tricortical graft did not differ with respect to the source – allograft or autograft. Although the iliac crest is a reliable source of bone, this technique is associated with developing degenerative changes at the recipient site and sometimes pain at the donor site [74]. Allogeneic grafts are designed to reduce these disadvantages [75]. Although the concern of early resorption and inadequate osseointegration of the allograft arises, clinical data show excellent functional results, low recurrence rates, and high osseointegration.

Ernstbrunner analyzed the position of a free tricortical graft in glenoid defect reconstruction, comparing arthroscopic and open surgical technique in two groups of 20 patients. In the arthroscopic group, a steeper angle of impact of the graft and a significantly greater medial offset of the graft were found compared to the open technique. The advantages of the arthroscopic technique are not directly related to the position of the graft and the reconstruction of the glenoid defect. They are rather the general advantages of arthroscopy: lower risk of infection, faster rehabilitation, cosmetics and last but not least - less trauma to the subscapularis muscle. This technique prevents the hypotrophy and fatty degeneration seen with the open technique [76].

A comparative detailed analysis by Moroder on the most used techniques for bone augmentation, namely coracoid transfer (Latarjet) and free tricortical iliac graft (Eden-Hybinette/ (ICBGT)) shows the lack of a significant advantage of each of the mentioned techniques [77]. At one-year follow-up, no statistically significant difference was observed in the functional scores - WOSI, SSV, ASOSS and Rowe. Regarding the range of motion (at 0° and 90° abduction), again no significant difference was reported except for internal rotation in favor of the free tricortical graft. A probable reason for this is the permanent structural splitting of the subscapularis muscle from the common tendon of the coracoid (the so-called conjoined tendon). Biomechanical studies of the sling effect with the Latarjet technique show a significant loss of total rotation at 90° abduction, compared with the free tricortical graft technique.

CT analysis shows another important feature of the free bone graft technique. This is the improved bony augmentation of the glenoid defect in the sense of increased total surface area, reduced volume of the defect, increased diameter and depth of the glenoid fossa. This is partly due to the purely anatomical limitation of the native coracoid process. Conversely, the size of the free graft is determined by the extent of the defect and the surgeon's technical performance [77].

Another interesting fact from Moroder's study is the absence of a statistically significant difference in the isokinetics of the patients after one of these techniques. The difference in this parameter was maintained in favor of the free tricortical graft within 1 year after surgery. At the end of the follow-up, the results were identical.

3.3 Tibial auto/allograft

Wong and Urquhart published an arthroscopic technique for glenoid augmentation using a distal tibial allograft that avoids damage to the subscapularis muscle and therefore allows for faster recovery [78]. The technique is based on the classic Bankart arthroscopic technique. Only one additional medial portal (Halifax portal) is required, which is done using an inside-out technique to avoid injury to the neuro-vascular structures. This is done through the posterior working portal, directed superiorly over the subscapularis muscle and laterally from the conjoined tendon of the coracoid - through the deltopectoral interval. Because the portal is inside-out, it is parallel to the glenoid surface and reproducible for safe passage of the graft.

Amar presents in his series the positives of arthroscopic reconstruction with tibial allograft and short-term CT results [79]. The technique appears to reduce musculocutaneous and axillary nerve injuries because the insertion of the subscapularis muscle remains intact. Placement of the additional Halifax portal using an inside-out technique allows identification of the aforementioned two structures, thereby protecting them from injury. With this technique, the Halifax portal was found to be an average of 4 cm from the above neural structures. In the Amar study, 18 patients (58%) had either less than 50% or more than 50% graft resorption. However, none of these patients with documented bone resorption reported residual shoulder instability [79]. Most importantly, even in the case of greater than 50% resorption, there was an increase in sagittal glenoid diameter of an average of 5.1 mm, which has been shown to be sufficient for clinical stability of the shoulder. This is probably due to the larger size of the graft that was used compared to the physiological size of the defect.

3.4 Graft remodeling

Coracoid transfer (Latarjet), free tricortical iliac graft (ICBGT), and distal tibial transfer are considered the most common operative techniques for bone augmentation [71, 77, 80].

The biomechanical effect of these techniques has been repeatedly demonstrated on cadavers [81, 82]. Over time, remodeling processes lead to changes in the articulating glenoid surface diameter, version, and depth after bony reconstruction. These processes vary between individual patients, depending on the degree of exercise, and are directly related to Wolff's law [83].

Sigrist analyzed the effectiveness of free tricortical graft (ICBGT) in restoring the glenoid surface and bone remodeling after this technique - both autograft and allograft. According to the author, the degree of remodeling also affects the degree of stability (stability ratio/SR), and increased retroversion leads to increased stability (SR) [84]. Proportional to Wolf's law, areas with less mechanical stimulation show greater bone resorption and remodeling. Conversely, at the positions where the bone is subjected to loading - 2′-4′ o'clock, there is a lack of bone resorption, increased glenoid diameter and depth [85]. This also supports the benefits of autologous bone transfer from a biomechanical and morphological perspective. In his study, Sigrist reported statistically greater residual bone defects with the use of allograft. Increased bone resorption in allografts has also been reported in other series. The likely cause of the excessive bone resorption is the lack of cellular recolonization and vascularization of the allograft. The use of fresh-frozen allografts instead of lyophilized ones improves the results of allograft bone augmentation. For example, distal tibial allografts show excellent resistance to bone resorption [86]. Autologous bone transfer (auto-ICBGT) increases the biomechanical stability of the shoulder not only immediately postoperatively, but also in the long-term aspect. Due to their rapid osteolysis, all allogeneic bone grafts suffer from the lack of improvement in stability and increase in bone parameters of the glenoid - width, depth, version, etc.

In 2020 Bois published a consensus of members of the three largest orthopedic associations in the United States regarding the approach and therapeutic options for bony defects in anterior shoulder instability [87]. With regard to known risk factors associated with critical bone loss, consensus among subspecialties has been reached that the total number of shoulder dislocations directly influences the magnitude of bone loss. In 2019, Dickens et al. conducted a study of athletes over a 4-year period to determine the amount of glenoid bone loss associated with first dislocation and recurrent instability. After a first dislocation, the mean loss of glenoid width was 6.8%, increasing to 22.8% after a second episode of instability [88]. In Gottschalk's 2017 systematic review on studies reporting percentage loss of glenoid width, 23.6% of cases had glenoid width loss between 10% and 25% [89].

Furthermore, in a prospective multicenter cohort study, Rugg showed that first-time dislocator patients were less likely to have bone loss or biceps pathology and the treatment procedure of choice was arthroscopic capsulolabral repair. Recurrent dislocations are more likely to require an open Latarjet to address critical bone loss [90]. These studies support a link between recurrent instability and the creation of critical bone loss. Some autors demonstrated in a prospective cohort study that male patients <25 years of age had a 78% chance of recurrent instability within 2 years of injury, which increased to 85% within 5 years of the initial injury when patients were treated nonoperatively [90].

Regarding the treatment of combined critical bipolar bone loss and previous failed Bankart soft tissue stabilization, Latarjet transfer is unanimous. For revision caces in which glenoid bone loss is maintained constant, and humerus loss is corrected, again the recommendation is for Latarjet stabilization.

Although other bone augmentation techniques were indicated as potential options for study participants, Latarjet stabilization was the most commonly preferred bone procedure for correction of bone deficiency. In a recent systematic review (13 studies, 845 shoulders) analyzing long-term outcomes after Latarjet stabilization, Hurley found an overall high rate of return to sport (84.9%) and a low rate of recurrence of instability (8.5%) [91]. The return-to-sport and recurrent instability rates found by Hurley remain significantly better than those reported after arthroscopic Bankart [92].

The general understanding based on the consensus is that, the choice for bone augmentation in the presence of bipolar bone loss is the augmentation of the glenoid defect, at the expense of the size of the Hill-Sachs defect, which appears to be secondary [87].

The cut-off value for determining the optimal surgical treatment in the presence of bipolar bone loss remains controversial. In Rossi's study, 90.1% of the experts agreed that in cases where the glenoid bone deficit was greater than 20%, the reconstruction of the glenoid bone loss should be with bone augmentation; in the presence of an acute bony Bankart lesion, fixation of the fragment can be performed arthroscopically using anchors [93].

Regarding graft type, the general statement of the panel is that any of the available options (coracoid, tricortical iliac graft, distal clavicle or distal tibia) is appropriate. However, in cases where the defect is very severe, the best option is to use a tricortical iliac graft. Some recent studies have reported that the critical cutoff value of glenoid bone loss should be lower than 20%. Shaha evaluated the clinical outcomes and recurrence rates among 72 patients with anterior shoulder instability divided into groups according to the size of the bony defects. It suggests that a glenoid bone defect greater than 13.5% will result in a clinically significant reduction in functional instability scores (WOSI), even in patients without postoperative recurrence [11].

4. Conclusion

Glenoid bone deficiency is major problem after shoulder dislocation and main reason for shoulder instability. Precise diagnosis and measurement ot this defect is essential for proper treatment. Bone augmetation techniques are treatment options for gainig stable joint and preventing reccurency. Open teshniques are still more popular because their simplicity, reliability and effectiveness. Atrhroscopic variants of those open techiques are becoming more popular, but still require technical support, surgeon experience and bigger expenses.

Author details

Svetoslav Dobrilov
University Hospital "St. Marina", Varna, Bulgaria

*Address all correspondence to: svetlyo_d@yahoo.com

References

[1] Zacchilli MA, Owens BD. Epidemiology of shoulder dislocations presenting to emergency departments in the United States. The Journal of Bone and Joint Surgery. American Volume. 2010;**92**(3):542-549

[2] Hovelius L, Olofsson A, Sandstrom B, Augustini BG, Krantz L, Fredin H, et al. Nonoperative treatment of primary anterior shoulder dislocation in patients forty years of age and younger. A prospective twenty-five-year follow-up. The Journal of Bone and Joint Surgery. American Volume. 2008;**90**(5):945-952

[3] Roberts SB, Beattie N, McNiven ND, Robinson CM. The natural history of primary anterior dislocation of the glenohumeral joint in adolescence. Bone Joint Journal. 2015;**97-B, 4**:520-526

[4] Spatschil A, Landsiedl F, Anderl W, et al. Posttraumatic anterior-inferior instability of the shoulder: Arthroscopic findings and clinical correlations. Archives of Orthopaedic and Trauma Surgery. 2005;**11**:1-6

[5] Burkhart SS, De Beer JF. Traumatic glenohumeral bone defects and their relationship to failure of arthroscopic Bankart repairs: Significance of the inverted-pear glenoid and the humeral engaging hill–Sachs lesion. Arthroscopy. 2000;**16**:677-694

[6] Su F, Kowalczuk M, Ikpe S, Lee H, Sabzevari S, Lin A. Risk factors for failure of arthroscopic revision anterior shoulder stabilization. The Journal of Bone and Joint Surgery. American Volume. 2018;**100**(15):1319-1312

[7] Arce G, Shea KP. Outcomes Scores for Shoulder Instability and Rotator Cuff Disease. In: Shoulder Concepts 2013: Consensus and Concerns. Berlin, Heidelberg: Springer; 2013. DOI: 10.1007/978-3-642-38097-6_6

[8] Boileau P, Villalba M, Hery JY, Balg F, Ahrens P, et al. Risk factors for recurrence of shoulder instability after arthroscopic Bankart repair. The Journal of Bone and Joint Surgery. American Volume. 2006;**88**:1755-1763

[9] Nakagawa S, Ozaki R, Take Y, et al. Relationship between glenoid defects and hill-Sachs lesions in shoulders with traumatic anterior shoulder instability. The American Journal of Sports Medicine. 2015;**43**:2763-2773

[10] Carrazzone OL, Tamaoki MJ, Ambra LF, Neto NA, Matsumoto MH, et al. Prevalence of lesions associated with traumatic recurrent shoulder dislocation. Revista Brasileira de Ortopedia. 2011;**46**:281-287. DOI: 10.1016/S2255-4971(15)30196-8

[11] Shaha JS, Cook JB, Song DJ, Rowles DJ, Bottoni CR, et al. Redefining “critical” bone loss in shoulder instability: Functional outcomes worsen with “subcritical” bone loss. The American Journal of Sports Medicine. 2015;**43**:1719-1725

[12] Piasecki DP, Verma NN, Romeo AA, Levine WN, Bach BR Jr, et al. Glenoid bone deficiency in recurrent anterior shoulder instability: Diagnosis and management. The Journal of the American Academy of Orthopaedic Surgeons. 2009;**17**:482-493

[13] Edwards TB, Boulahia A, Walch G. Radiographic analysis of bone defects in chronic anterior shoulder instability. Arthroscopy. 2003;**19**:732-773

[14] Sugaya H, Moriishi J, Kanisawa I, Tsuchiya A. Arthroscopic

osseous Bankart repair for chronic recurrent traumatic anterior glenohumeral instability. Journal Bone Joint Surgery America. 2005;**87**:1752-1760

[15] Boileau P, Bicknell RT, El Fegoun AB. Chuinard C arthroscopic Bristow procedure for anterior instability in shoulders with a stretched or deficient capsule: The 'belt-and-suspenders' operative technique and preliminary results. Arthroscopy. 2007;**23**:593-601

[16] Chuang TY, Adam CR, Burkhart SS. Use of preoperative three-dimensional computed tomography to quantify glenoid bone loss in shoulder instability. Arthroscopy. 2008;**24**:376-373

[17] Bigliani LU, Newton PM, Steinmann SP, et al. Glenoid rim lesions associated with recurrent anterior dislocation of the shoulder. The American Journal of Sports Medicine. 1998;**26**:41-455

[18] Griffith J, Antonio G, Tong C, Ming C. Anterior shoulder dislocation: Quantification of glenoid bone loss with CT. American Journal of Radiology. 2003;**180**:1423-1430

[19] Itoi E, Lee SB, Amrami KK, et al. Quantitative assessment of classic anteroinferior bony Bankart lesions by radiography and computed tomography. The American Journal of Sports Medicine. 2003;**31**:112-118

[20] Saito H, Itoi E, Sugaya H, et al. Location of the glenoid defect in shoulders with recurrent anterior dislocation. The American Journal of Sports Medicine. 2005;**33**:889-893

[21] Yamamoto N, Itoi E, Abe H, et al. Contact between the glenoid and the humeral head in abduction, external rotation, and horizontal extension: A new concept of glenoid track. Journal of Shoulder and Elbow Surgery. 2007;**16**:649-656.15

[22] Iannotti JP, Gabriel JP, Schneck SL, et al. The normal glenohumeral relationships: An anatomic study of one hundred and forty shoulders. The Journal of Bone and Joint Surgery. American Volume. 1992;**74**:491-500

[23] De Wilde LF, Berghs BM, Audenaert E, Sys G, Van Maele GO, Barbaix E. About the variability of the shape of the glenoid cavity. Surgical and Radiologic Anatomy. 2004;**26**:54-59

[24] Aigner F, Longato S, Fritsch H, Kralinger F. Anatomical considerations regarding the "bare spot" of the glenoid cavity. Surgical and Radiologic Anatomy. 2004;**26**:308-311

[25] Huijsmans PE, Haen PS, Kidd M, Dhert WJ, van der Hulst VP, et al. Quantification of a glenoid defect with three-dimensional computed tomography and magnetic resonance imaging: A cadaveric study. Journal of Shoulder and Elbow Surgery. 2007;**16**:803-809

[26] Owens BD, Nelson BJ, Duffey ML, et al. Pathoanatomy of first time, traumatic, anterior glenohumeral subluxation events. Journal of Bone and Joint Surgery. 2010;**92**(7):1605-1611

[27] Guity MR, Akhlaghpour S, Yousefian R. Determination of prevalence of glenoid bony lesions after recurrent anterior shoulder dislocation using the 3-D CT scan. Medical Journal of the Islamic Republic of Iran. 2014;**28**:20

[28] Itoi E, Lee SB, Berglund LJ, et al. The effect of a glenoid defecton anteroinferior stability of the shoulder after Bankart repair: A cadaveric study.

The Journal of Bone and Joint Surgery. American Volume. 2000;**82**:35-46

[29] Omori Y, Yamamoto N, Koishi H, et al. Glenoid track in live shoulders using 3D MRI motion analysis. In: Read at 37th Annual Meeting. Sendai: Japan Shoulder Society; 2010

[30] Ozaki R, Nakagawa S, Mizuno N, et al. Hill-Sachs lesions in shoulders with traumatic anterior instability: Evaluation using computed tomography with 3-dimensional reconstruction. The American Journal of Sports Medicine. 2014;**42**:2597-2605

[31] Nakagawa S, Hanai H, Mae T, et al. Bipolar bone loss in male athletes with traumatic anterior instability: An examiation using a new scoring system. Orthopaedic Journal of Sports Medicine. 2018;**6**(7):232596711878242

[32] Nakagawa S, Iuchi R, Hanai H. The development process of bipolar bone defects from primary to recurrent instability in shoulders with traumatic anterior instability. The American Journal of Sports Medicine. Mar 2019;**47**(3):695-703

[33] Randelli P, Ragone V, Carminati S, Cabitza P. Risk factorsfor recurrence after Bankart repair a systematic review. Knee Surgery, Sports Traumatology, Arthroscopy. 2012;**20**:2129-2138

[34] Porcellini G, Campi F, Pegreffi F, Castagna A, Paladini P. Predisposing factors for recurrent shoulder dislocation after arthroscopic treatment. The Journal of Bone and Joint Surgery. American Volume. 2009;**91**(11):2537-2542

[35] Imhoff AB, Ansah P, Tischer T, Reiter C, Bartl C, Hench M, et al. Arthroscopic repair of anterior-inferior glenohumeral instability using a portal at the 5:30-o'clock position: Analysis of the effects of age, fixation method, and concomitant shoulder injury on surgical outcomes. The American Journal of Sports Medicine. 2010;**38**(9):1795-1803

[36] Nakagawa S, Ozaki R, Take Y, et al. Enlargement of glenoid defects in traumatic anterior shoulder instability: Influence of the number of recurrences and type of sports. Orthopaedic Journal of Sports Medicine. 2014;**2**(4):2325967114529920

[37] Flinkkila T, Hyvonen P, Ohtonen P. Leppilahti J arthroscopic Bankart repair: Results and risk factors of recurrence of instability. Knee Surgery, Sports Traumatology, Arthroscopy. 2010;**18**(12):1752-1758

[38] Pansard E, Klouche S, Billot N, Rousselin B, Kraus TM, et al. Reliability and validity assessment of a glenoid bone loss measurement using the Bernageau profile view in chronic anterior shoulder instability. Journal of Shoulder and Elbow Surgery. 2013;**22**:1193-1198

[39] Huysmans E, Haen P, Kidd M. The shape of the inferior part of the glenoid: A cadaveric study. Journal of Shoulder and Elbow Surgery. 2006;**15**(6):759-761

[40] Sugaya H, Moriishi J, Dohi M. Glenoid rim morphology inrecurrent anterior glenohumeral instability. The Journal of Bone and Joint Surgery. American Volume. 2003;**85**:878-884

[41] Verweij L, Schuit A. Accuracy of currently available methods in quantifying anterior glenoid bone loss: Controversy regarding gold standard – A systematic review. Arthroscopy: The Journal of Arthroscopic and Related Surgery. Aug 2020;**36**(8):2295-2313

[42] Baudi P, Righi P, Bolognesi D, Rivetta S, Rossi Urtoler E, et al. How to identify and calculate glenoid bone

deficit. La Chirurgia degli organi di movimento. 2005;**90**:145-152

[43] Magarelli N, Milano G, Baudi P, Santagada DA, Righi P, et al. Comparison between 2D and 3D computed tomography evaluation of glenoid bone defect in unilateral anterior Gleno-humeral instability. La Radiologia Medica. 2012;**117**:102-111

[44] Loppini M, Delle Rose G, Borroni M, Morenghi E, Pitino D, et al. Is the instability severity index score a valid tool for predicting failure after primary arthroscopic stabilization for anterior Glenohumeral instability? Arthroscopy. 2019;**35**:361-366

[45] Bakshi NK, Cibulas GA, Sekiya JK, Bedi A. A clinical comparison of linear- and surface area-based methods of measuring glenoid bone loss. The American Journal of Sports Medicine. 2018;**46**:2472-2477

[46] Provencher MT, Bhatia S, Ghodadra NS, Grumet RC, Bach BR Jr, et al. Recurrent shoulder instability: Current concepts for evaluation and management of glenoid bone loss. The Journal of Bone and Joint Surgery. American Volume. 2010;**92**(Suppl. 2): 133-151

[47] Bhatia S, Saigal A, Frank RM, Bach BR Jr, Cole BJ, et al. Glenoid diameter is an inaccurate method for percent glenoid bone loss quantification: Analysis and techniques for improved accuracy. Arthroscopy. 2015;**31**:608-614

[48] Bois AJ, Fening SD, Polster J, Jones MH, Miniaci A. Quantifying glenoid bone loss in anterior shoulder instability: Reliability and accuracy of 2-dimensional and 3-dimensional computed tomography measurement techniques. The American Journal of Sports Medicine. 2012;**40**:2569-2577

[49] Moroder P, Plachel F, Huettner A, Ernstbrunner L, Minkus M, et al. The effect of scapula tilt and best-fit circle placement when measuring glenoid bone loss in shoulder instability patients. Arthroscopy. 2018;**34**:398-404

[50] Burkhart SS, Debeer JF, Tehrany AM, Parten PM. Quantifying glenoid bone loss arthroscopically in shoulder instability. Arthroscopy. 2002;**18**:488-491

[51] Hamamoto JT, Leroux T, Chahla J, Bhatia S, Higgins JD, et al. Assessment and evaluation of glenoid bone loss. Arthroscopy Techniques. 2016;**5**:e947-e951

[52] Shin SJ, Jun BJ, Koh YW, McGarry MH, Lee TQ. Estimation of anterior glenoid bone loss area using the ratio of bone defect length to the distance from posterior glenoid rim to the Centre of the glenoid. Knee Surgery, Sports Traumatology, Arthroscopy. 2018;**26**:48-55

[53] Miyatake K, Takeda Y, Fujii K, Takasago T, Iwame T. Validity of arthroscopic measurement of glenoid bone loss using the bare spot. Open access Journal of Sports Medicine. 2014;**5**:37-42

[54] Walter WR, Samim M, LaPolla FWZ, Gyftopoulos S. Imaging quantification of glenoid bone loss in patients with glenohumeral instability: A systematic review. American Journal of Roentgenology. May 2019;**212**(5):1096-1105

[55] Balg F, Boileau P. The instability severity index score. A simple pre-operative score to select patients for arthroscopic or open shoulder stabilisation. Journal of Bone and Joint Surgery. British Volume (London). 2007;**89**:1470-1477

[56] Thomazeau H, Langlais T, Hardy A, Curado J, Herisson O, et al. Long-621

term, prospective, Multicenter study of isolated Bankart repair for a patient selection method based on the instability severity index score. The American Journal of Sports Medicine. Apr 2019;**47**(5):1057-1061

[57] Taverna E, D'Ambrosi R. Arthroscopic Bone Graft Procedure for Anterior Inferior Glenohumeral Instability. Arthroscopy Techniques. 2014;**3**(6):e653-ee66

[58] Bhatia S, Frank RM, Ghodadra NS, Hsu AR, Romeo AA, Bach BR, et al. The outcomes and surgical techniques of the Latarjet procedure. Arthroscopy. 2014;**30**:227-235

[59] Giles J, Degen R. The Bristow and Latarjet procedures: Why these techniques should not Be considered synonymous. JBJS. 2014;**16**(96):1340-1348

[60] Hurley ET, Lim Fat D, Farrington SK, Mullett H. Open versus arthroscopic latarjet procedure for anterior shoulder instability: A sistematic review and meta-analysis. The American Journal of Sports Medicine. 2019;**47**:1248-1253

[61] Marion B, Klouche S, Deranlot J, Bauer T, Nourissat G, Hardy P. A prospective comparative study of arthroscopic versus mini-open Latarjet procedure with a minimum 2-year follow-up. Arthroscopy. 2016;**33**(2):269-277

[62] Nourissat G, Neyton L, Metais P, et al. Functional outcomes after open versus arthroscopic Latarjet procedure: A prospective comparative study. Orthopaedics & Traumatology, Surgery & Research. 2016;**102**(8):277-279

[63] Randelli P, Fossati C, Stoppani C, Evola FR, De Girolamo L. Open Latarjet versus arthroscopic Latarjet: Clinical results and cost analysis. Knee Surgery, Sports Traumatology, Arthroscopy. 2016;**24**(2):526-532

[64] Gupta A, Delaney R, Petkin K, Lafosse L. Complications of the Latarjet procedure. Current Reviews in Musculoskeletal Medicine. 2015;**8**:59-66

[65] Nourissat G, Delaroche C, Bouillet B, Doursounian L, Aim F. Optimization of bone-block positioning in the Bristow-Latarjet procedure: A biomechanical study. Orthopaedics & Traumatology, Surgery & Research. 2014;**100**:509-513

[66] Kany J, Flamand O, Grimberg J, et al. Arthroscopic Latarjet procedure: Is optimal positioning of the bone block and screws possible? A prospective computed tomography scan analysis. Journal of Shoulder and Elbow Surgery. 2016;**25**:69-77

[67] Kordasiewicz B, Małachowski K, Kicinski M, Chaberek S, Pomianowski S. Comparative study of open and arthroscopic coracoid transfer for shoulder anterior instability (Latarjet) clinical results at short term follow-up. International Orthopaedics. 2017;**41**:1023-1033

[68] Ali J, Altintas B, Pulatkan A. Open versus arthroscopic Latarjet procedure for the treatment of chronic anterior Glenohumeral instability with glenoid bone loss. Arthroscopy: The Journal of Arthroscopic and Related Surgery. 2020;**36**(4 April):940-949

[69] Galvin J, Zimmer Z, Prete A, Warner JJP. The open Eden-Hybinette procedure for Reurrent anterior shoulder instability with glenoid bone loss. Operative Techniques in Sports Medicine. 2019;**27**(2):95-101

[70] Warner JJ, Gill TJ, O'Hollerhan JD, et al. Anatomical glenoid reconstruction for recurrent anterior glenohumeral

instability with glenoid deficiency using an autogenous tricortical iliac crest bone graft. The American Journal of Sports Medicine. 2006;**34**:205-212

[71] Kraus N, Amphansap T, Gerhardt C, Scheibel M. Arthroscopic anatomic glenoid reconstruction using an autologous iliac crest bone grafting technique. Journal of Shoulder and Elbow Surgery. 2014;**23**:1700-1708

[72] Giannakos A, Vezeridis PS, Schwartz DG, et al. All-arthroscopic revision Eden-Hybinette procedure for failed instability surgery: Technique and preliminary results. Arthroscopy. 2017;**33**:39-48

[73] Malahias M, Chytas D, Raoulis V. Iliac crest bone grafting for the Management of Anterior Shoulder Instability in patients with glenoid bone loss: A systematic review of contemporary literature. Sports Medicine - Open. 2020;**6**:12

[74] Moroder P, Blocher M, Auffarth A, et al. Clinical and computed tomography radiologic outcome after bony glenoid augmentation in recurrent anterior shoulder instability without significant glenoid bone loss. Journal of Shoulder and Elbow Surgery. 2014;**23**(3):420-426.44

[75] Willemot LB, Elhassan BT, Verborgt O. Bony reconstruction of the anterior glenoid rim. The Journal of the American Academy of Orthopaedic Surgeons. 2018;**26**(10):e207-e218

[76] Ernstbrunner L, Plachel P, Heuberer P. Arthroscopic versus open iliac crest bone grafting in recurrent anterior shoulder instability with glenoid bone loss: A computed Tomographye based quantitative assessment. Arthroscopy: The Journal of Arthroscopic and Related Surgery. 2018;**34**(2):352-359

[77] Moroder P, Schulz E, Wierer G. Neer award 2019: Latarjet procedure vs. iliac crest bone graft transfer for treatment of anterior shoulder instability with glenoid bone loss: A prospective randomized trial. Journal of Shoulder and Elbow Surgery. 2019;**28**:1298-1307

[78] Wong IH, Urquhart N. Arthroscopic anatomic glenoid reconstruction without subscapularis split. Arthroscopy Techniques. 2015;**4**(5):e449-e456

[79] Amar E, Konstantinidis G, Coady C, Wong IH. Arthroscopic treatment of shoulder instability with glenoid bone loss using distal tibial allograft augmentation: Safety profile and short-term radiological outcomes. Orthopaedic Journal of Sports Medicine. 2018;**6**(5):1-6

[80] Lafosse L, Lejeune E, Bouchard A, et al. The arthroscopic Latarjet procedure for the treatment of anterior shoulder instability. Arthroscopy. 2007;**23**(1242):e1-e5

[81] Boons HW, Giles JW, Elkinson I, Johnson JA, Athwal GS. Classic versus congruent coracoid positioning during the Latarjet procedure: An in vitro biomechanical comparison. Arthroscopy. 2013;**29**(2):309-331

[82] Giles JW, Boons HW, Elkinson I, et al. Does the dynamic sling effect of the Latarjet procedure improve shoulder stability? A biomechanical evaluation. Journal of Shoulder and Elbow Surgery. 2013;**22**(6):821-827

[83] Moroder P, Hitzl W, Tauber M, Hoffelner T, Resch H, Auffarth A. Effect of anatomic bone grafting in post-traumatic recurrent anterior shoulder instability on glenoid morphology. Journal of Shoulder and Elbow Surgery. 2013;**22**(11):1522-1529

[84] Sigrist B, Ferguson S, Boehmc E. The biomechanical effect of bone grafting

and bone graft Remodeling in patients with anterior shoulder instability. The American Journal of Sports Medicine. Jul 2020;**48**(8):1857-1864

[85] Haas M, Plachel F, Wierer G, et al. Glenoid morphology is associated with the development of instability arthropathy. Journal of Shoulder and Elbow Surgery. 2019;**28**(5):893-899

[86] Provencher MT, Frank RM, Golijanin P, et al. Distal tibia allograft glenoid reconstruction in recurrent anterior shoulder instability: Clinical and radiographic outcomes. Arthroscopy. 2017;**33**(5):891-897

[87] Bois A, Mayer M, Fening S. Management of bone loss in recurrent traumatic anterior shoulder instability: A survey of north American surgeons. JSES International. 26 May 2020;**4**(3):574-583

[88] Dickens JF, Slaven SE, Cameron KL, Pickett AM, Posner M, Campbell SE, et al. Prospective evaluation of glenoid bone loss after first-time and recurrent anterior glenohumeral instability events. The American Journal of Sports Medicine. 2019;**47**:1082e9

[89] Gottschalk LJ IV, Bois AJ, Shelby MA, Miniaci A, Jones MH. Mean glenoid defect size and location associated with anterior shoulder instability: A systematic review. Orthopaedic Journal of Sports Medicine. 2017;**5**:2325967116676269

[90] Rugg CM, Hettrich CM, Ortiz S, Wolf BR, Group MSI, Zhang AL. Surgical stabilization for first-time shoulder dislocators: A multicenter analysis. Journal of Shoulder and Elbow Surgery. 2018;**27**:674e85

[91] Hurley ET, Jamal MS, Ali ZS, Montgomery C, Pauzenberger L, Mullett H. Longterm outcomes of the Latarjet procedure for anterior shoulder instability: A systematic review of studies at 10-year follow-up. Journal of Shoulder and Elbow Surgery. 2019;**28**:e33e9

[92] Zimmermann SM, Scheyerer MJ, Farshad M, Catanzaro S, Rahm S, Gerber C. Long-term restoration of anterior shoulder stability: A retrospective analysis of arthroscopic Bankart repair versus open Latarjet procedure. The Journal of Bone and Joint Surgery. American Volume. 2016;**98**:1954e61

[93] Rossi L. et al. Evaluation and Management of Glenohumeral Instability with Associated Bone Loss: An expert consensus statement using the modified Delphi technique, Arthroscopy: The Journal of Arthroscopic and Related Surgery. 2021;37(6):1719-1728

Chapter 3

Arthroscopic Assisted versus Open Reduction and Internal Fixation of Greater Tuberosity Fractures of the Proximal Humerus

Raquel Guitián-Montes, Samer Amhaz-Escanlar, Alberto Jorge-Mora and Ana Carolina Presas-Presas

Abstract

Throughout this chapter, we will discuss the treatment of greater tuberosity fractures of the proximal humerus. Greater tuberosity fractures are common, and an increase is expected due to population aging. We can address these fractures in different ways to restore the anatomy and function of the patient, but surgery is usually selected for displaced fractures. The surgical approach remains unclear, and few data can guide surgeons in choosing one technique or another. We will discuss open versus less invasive and arthroscopic repair techniques for fractures of the greater tuberosity of the humerus, and we will try to underline the advantages and cons of each method and describe the evidence around each surgical technique. We will also include some tips and tricks that may be helpful to orthopedic surgeons to achieve an optimal outcome.

Keywords: arthroscopy, greater tuberosity fractures, shoulder, double-row suture, proximal humerus

1. Introduction

Isolated, more significant tuberosity fractures account for up to 20% of all proximal humeral fractures [1–3]. Proximal humerus fractures are more common in elderly female patients with poor bone quality following low-energy trauma. Women are affected three times more often than men. In contrast, in younger patients, greater tuberosity (GT) fractures usually occur in males following high-velocity trauma [4].

The proximal humerus, a critical upper limb component, possesses intricate anatomical, osteomuscular, vascular, and nervous structures that collectively contribute to its functionality and clinical significance. This region encompasses the humeral head, anatomical neck, greater and lesser tubercles, and adjacent soft tissues, all intricately interacting to enable a wide range of upper limb movements and maintain shoulder stability. A comprehensive understanding of the proximal humerus's osteomuscular, vascular, and nervous anatomy is essential for medical professionals involved in clinical assessment, surgical interventions, and rehabilitative strategies.

Numerous studies have explored the multifaceted anatomy of the proximal humerus. Anatomically, the humeral head articulates with the glenoid fossa of the scapula, forming the glenohumeral joint. This complex joint relies on a delicate balance of osteological structures, such as the articular surfaces and the anatomical neck, to ensure joint congruency and proper movement mechanics. Meanwhile, the greater and lesser tubercles are attachment sites for vital muscles, including the rotator cuff, contributing to the intricate dynamics of shoulder movement and stability.

Vascular supply to the proximal humerus is a vital aspect often explored in anatomical and clinical literature. Studies by Le Minor et al. [5] highlight the branching patterns of the humeral circumflex arteries, which are essential for nourishing the bone and surrounding tissues. A crucial aspect often investigated in anatomical studies is vascular supply to the greater tuberosity. Research by Iacobellis et al. [6] and Basat et al. [7] elucidates the vascularization patterns of the humeral tuberosities, including the trochiter, through angiographic studies. Understanding the blood supply to this region is crucial for surgical procedures involving the proximal humerus, as compromised blood flow can impact bone healing and tissue recovery.

The intricate neural network within the proximal humerus region has been extensively studied. Research by Standring et al. [8] emphasizes the role of the axillary and suprascapular nerves in innervating the muscles and transmitting sensory information from the shoulder region. Understanding nerve pathways is crucial in clinical settings to diagnose nerve-related issues, especially posttraumatic or iatrogenic injuries.

One must account for the forces that cause deformation due to the contraction of the rotator cuff (RC) muscles when deciding on the best surgical fixation approach for fractures involving the greater tubercle (GT). The supraspinatus, infraspinatus, and teres minor muscles all attach to the GT, and the combined effects of their forces are pivotal in maintaining proper shoulder function. Given the nature of these insertions, the direction of displacement can be anticipated. Most GT fractures involved the supraspinatus and infraspinatus facets, leading to superior and posterior GT displacement. The posterior displacement is difficult to measure because it is often underestimated and can lead to clinical impingement [2].

In the case of a comminuted fracture of the greater tubercle (GT), it is possible to observe two distinct fragments displaced in different directions. One fragment may be displaced in a superomedial direction, connected to the supraspinatus tendon, while another fragment may be displaced in a posteromedial direction, linked to the infraspinatus tendon [3].

The greater and lesser tuberosities receive small perforators from the anterior and posterior circumflex arteries. In addition, circumflex arteries and the nearby thoracoacromial, supra, and subscapular arteries are also anastomosed numerous times extraosseously. This vascular network explains why isolated fractures of the tuberosity rarely result in osteonecrosis of the humeral head [2, 9].

Most fractures of the greater tuberosity of the humerus can be satisfactorily treated non-surgically [10]. It should be noted that conservative treatment does not imply abandoning the lesion but will require close and serial follow-up with a rehabilitation program that restores function and mobility. Displaced fractures have been treated with various surgical methods, including open or percutaneous reduction and internal fixation (ORIF) and arthroscopically assisted fixation. The choice of fixation and approach is influenced by the patient's specific circumstances and the fracture's type, morphology, and characteristics [2].

Standard radiographs are typically used to diagnose these injuries, which usually present as acute shoulder pain with a decreased range of motion. In most cases, computed tomography (CT) is recommended because the evaluation of a 3D structure as the greater tuberosity and its position is not easily determined with simple X-rays. Mainly, it is advantageous when the fracture pattern cannot be adequately defined, and displacement and morphology fracture fragment morphology remain unclear [2, 3]. That can affect the surgical approach, technique, and selection of the implant. CT scans are also helpful for obese patients. That's why CT scans with coronal and sagittal plane reconstructions are being obtained in the emergency room setting with increasing frequency. However, a good quality complete shoulder radiographic series should preclude obtaining a CT scan in most cases.

Ultrasonography and even magnetic resonance imaging may be helpful, especially in fractures associated with instability.

Most authors agreed that surgical treatment of isolated GT fractures is indicated in patients with a displacement of 5 mm or more. Still, there is a trend to be more aggressive in this limit. Some authors suggest that patients with as little as 3 mm of superior displacement may benefit from surgical reduction and fixation in active [10]. Patients with posterior-superior GT displacement had significantly worse outcomes than those with anterior-inferior or anterior-superior GT displacement. It is unclear, though, how much posterior GT displacement is "acceptable" [3].

With a longer life expectancy and increased physical activity in all age groups, isolated tuberosity fractures of the proximal humeral are expected to rise [2]. For this reason, orthopedic surgeons who treat shoulder trauma must manage different techniques to treat displaced greater tuberosity fractures to be applied in the indicated situation to optimize outcomes.

2. Evaluation

The greater tuberosity is a significant anatomical structure, and shoulder external rotation and abduction depend on its integrity. Greater tuberosity isolated fractures are frequently undetectable on initial radiographs because they are so subtle [11].

These patients arrive holding the injured extremity close to the axial skeleton. Ecchymosis may extend into the axilla and distally along the upper arm, and there is swelling around the upper shoulder, according to an examination. In the acute setting, it is challenging to distinguish tuberosity fracture from cuff pathology clinically; imaging tests are essential to make this critical distinction. Patients will not tolerate the cuff strength test against resistance in both scenarios. A complete neurovascular examination should be performed as nerve injuries occur in one-third of greater tuberosity fracture-dislocations, with full recovery in most cases after several months. In addition, there may also be accompanying glenohumeral dislocations, which must be reduced promptly.

Neurovascular assessment is mandatory. We should complete a global evaluation of the brachial plexus, but it is essential to address with care four nerves: the axillary, musculocutaneous, radial, and suprascapular nerves. The axillary nerve, originating from the posterior cord of the brachial plexus, innervates the deltoid and teres minor muscles. A meticulous assessment of the axillary nerve involves evaluating the range of motion of the shoulder joint and testing the strength of deltoid muscle contraction. Clinical examination techniques, such as the "empty can" test, aid in detecting potential axillary nerve injuries or impingements, often resulting from trauma or overuse. The musculocutaneous nerve, emerging from the lateral cord of the brachial plexus, innervates the biceps, brachial, and brachialis muscles and provides sensory innervation to the lateral forearm. During the examination, the motor function of the biceps brachii is assessed through resistance testing and evaluating the elbow flexion strength. Sensory assessment involves evaluating the sensory perception on the lateral forearm to detect any areas of hypoesthesia or altered sensation. Greater tuberosity fractures are frequently associated with glenohumeral dislocation; in these cases, the radial nerve is the second nerve affected in shoulder dislocations (12.8%) after the axillary nerve [12]. Functional implications are debilitating, including wrist and finger drops. Most palsies recur without treatment in 3 to 6 months, so recovery rates are high. An EMG should be done if there is not any improvement in function after 3 to 6 months. The suprascapular nerve, originating from the upper trunk of the brachial plexus, innervates the supraspinatus and infraspinatus muscles, contributing to shoulder movement and stability. Examination techniques may involve evaluating the strength of these muscles through resisted movements and assessing any potential muscle atrophy. Acute assessment is complicated due to the fracture, but continuous evaluation during follow-up is necessary. Advanced diagnostic tools, including electromyography (EMG) and nerve conduction studies, can provide valuable insights into these nerves' functionality and potential dysfunctions.

Additionally, imaging modalities such as magnetic resonance imaging (MRI) and ultrasound can assist in visualizing the nerves and surrounding structures, aiding in diagnosing nerve compressions, injuries, or pathologies. An urgent angiogram evaluation is necessary to determine whether vascular intervention is required in the presence of an expanding hematoma, the absence of proximal pulses, and the emergence of upper extremity neuropathy. Even so, vascular injuries in this type of fracture are uncommon.

Isolated fracture of the tuberosity may lead to concomitant rotator cuff tears, which may be the etiology of the patient's persistent discomfort after fracture union.

The initial technique to detect a fracture of the greater tuberosity of the humerus is plain x-rays. It is recommended to perform an AP view in external rotation and an AP view with a caudal inclination of 15° to define greater tuberosity displacement most accurately. In most situations, displacement is underestimated.

If the x-ray shows us an evident displacement of >5 mm, surgery can be considered based on the activity expectations of each patient. On images, where the degree of displacement is not evident or is borderline (3 to 5 mm), other diagnostic tests may be used, and CT is our gold standard.

If a fracture is suspected, but not identified on radiographs or with a borderline displacement, computed tomography (CT) or MRI may be obtained. MRI has the advantage of evaluating the rotator cuff, bone edema, and labral injuries. In some situations, ultrasound is being chosen as the evaluation modality in many centers when initial radiographs do not provide clear information because more experience is being gained by an increasing number of professionals and it is a non-invasive technique (PoCUS – Point of Care Ultrasound) [2, 11, 13].

The greater tuberosity is an important anatomic structure and its integrity is important for shoulder abduction and external rotation. Isolated fractures of the greater tuberosity are often subtle and may not be detected initially.

3. Surgical treatment

The goal of surgical treatment is to restore anatomy and allow early movement with stable fixation. The selection of an appropriate surgical technique and implant depends on the size of the fragment, the amount of displacement, the level of comminution, and the presence of osteoporosis.

Positioning of the patient is critical to improve visualization of the fragments and adequate implant placement for fixation, and most authors recommend the beach chair position (**Figure 1**) for both arthroscopic, open or percutaneous techniques, because it allows manipulation of the arm during the procedure, and it is easy to orient. Surgery may also be performed with minimal assistance with the aid of mechanical arm fixation devices such as assist arm. Although the position with which the surgeon is most comfortable and has more experience should be used, being the position in lateral decubitus with longitudinal traction of the affected extremity also valid (**Figure 2**).

The anesthesia used is a combination of general anesthesia and regional block for intraoperative pain control. If we selected arthroscopically assisted techniques, it is mandatory to optimize patient's blood pressure to minimize bleeding and facilitate visualization. The local use of adrenaline with a local anesthetic minimizes pain and facilitates the anesthesiologist blood pressure control.

3.1 Open reduction

Classically, open reduction and internal fixation have been selected for displaced greater tuberosity fractures. Theoretically, it allows a better visualization and facilitates reduction of the fragment with acceptable rates of union and low rates of complications, with good postoperative outcomes. We can choose between two approaches for this fixation, the deltopectoral approach, which is usually selected in those situations where we need to use a plate, and the transdeltoid approach which may be applied with a longitudinal incision or through a standard anterolateral approach [14, 15].

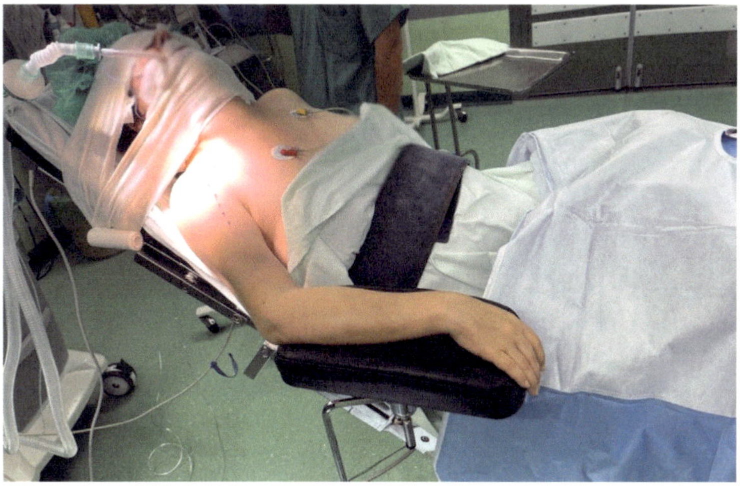

Figure 1.
Chair position.

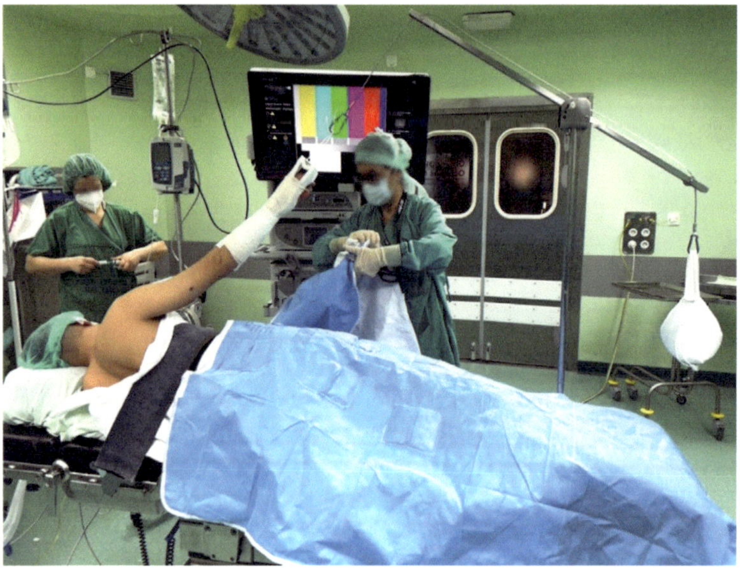

Figure 2.
Lateral decubitus with longitudinal traction.

Several fixation techniques have been described to achieve reduction and stabilization, including trans osseous sutures, locking plates with or without suture augmentation, and screw fixation via open or closed reduction. Each of these techniques is briefly described below.

Trans osseous sutures with non-absorbable sutures passing through the rotator cuff tendon are an option that has shown good effects in biomechanical studies compared to suture anchor techniques in the treatment of greater tuberosity fractures [16], being preferable in patients with poor bone quality. Trans osseous suture allows the fragment fixation obviating the need for a second surgery for implant removal [17].

Open reduction and internal fixation with locking plates combined or not with suture reinforcement are described as a very useful technique for the treatment of greater tuberosity fractures, especially in osteoporotic bone with big fragments [18, 19]. Open plate osteosynthesis provides accurate reduction under direct visualization, rigid fixation of the avulsed fragment, and early mobilization facilitating good functional outcomes, decreasing the possibility of reduction loosening and secondary displacement [20]. The preferred approach for plate fixation is the deltopectoral approach but recent studies have shown promising results with shorter plates that need smaller incisions for placement [14, 20]. This lower profile plates, not specific for this greater tuberosity fractures, have been described to avoid or reduce the complication associated with classic plates and maintaining the rates of union and functional recovery [20]. For these techniques, the use of an anterolateral approach has demonstrated non-inferior outcomes with less complications [21].

Al last, percutaneous fixation with cannulated screws with or without washers has the advantages of a minimally invasive technique, less intraoperative blood loss, shorter hospital stays, and fewer complications related to the incision [22, 23]. Despite this, a non-despicable rate of postoperative stiffness is reported in patients treated with this method [24]. The handicap to performing this minimally invasive technique is confirming anatomical reduction. It is not easy to achieve GT anatomical restoration by closed maneuvers, and in the case of using high compression techniques such as screws with a washer, we may generate a malposition due to overreduction by compression. Comminuted fractures and osteoporotic bones may make percutaneous screw fixation difficult, increasing the hazard of malreduction. In these cases, using devices such as percutaneous low-profile plates or classical plates through an open approach may be preferable [20].

3.2 Arthroscopic repair techniques

Arthroscopically assisted fixation has gained popularity because it brings the "best of both worlds". When we have a small or osteoporotic fragment, with comminution, we may reduce it under direct visualization in a way like the open technique and we can complete a less invasive fixation with a percutaneous technique. Arthroscopically techniques for rotator cuff tears increase the rigidity of the fixation and favor tension distribution to bone also in osteoporotic bone.

Multiple techniques have been described, but the most widespread and accepted by the authors is perhaps the arthroscopic double-row suture anchor fixation technique (ADSF).

With the patient under general anesthesia, the patient is positioned in the beach chair position. Next, a posterior portal is formed with 2 cm inferior and 2 cm medial to the posterolateral corner of the acromion [22]. An arthroscope is inserted through the posterior portal, and we perform a complete intraarticular examination as a diagnostic arthroscopy after irrigation of the hemarthroses caused by the fracture. Next, we create an anterior working portal through the rotator interval and treat any concurrent pathology found during the arthroscopic examination. The arthroscope is then advanced through the posterior portal to the subacromial space, and a working portal is established 2 cm lateral to the acromion's anterolateral corner [25–28]. All subacromial pathology is addressed currently.

We identify the fracture and with the help of a shaver and a burr, debridement is performed under the fracture bed at the humerus. This step also serves to create a bleeding bone surface conducive to healing. With the aid of an arthroscopic grasper and a probe, we reduce the fracture to its anatomical position. Then, correct fracture reduction is confirmed with fluoroscopy.

Next, a knotless self-reinforcing double-row repair is performed with four anchors (two medial anchors and two lateral anchors). In very large fragments, it may be necessary to add more anchors.

Through the anterolateral working portal, two medial anchors (one anteromedial and one posteromedial) loaded with suture tape are inserted into the articular margin of the humeral head, medial to the fracture bed. Maintaining a 15 mm gap between each medial anchor in the anteroposterior direction is recommended. The medial sutures are passed through the intact rotator cuff.

An arthroscopic forceps and suture passer are used to insert each end of the suture tape through the rotator cuff tendon and 3 to 5 mm medial to the bone fragment.

Next, we proceed to implant the lateral row of suture anchors that are placed similar to the medial anchors. The two anchors inserted lateral to the fracture bed are loaded with one limb of the suture tapes from each of the medial anchors, and the repair is completed by tying the sutures above the fracture fragment (**Figure 3**).

Under both direct arthroscopic visualization and fluoroscopy, the correct stability and reduction are confirmed in the passive range of motion of the shoulder. It is

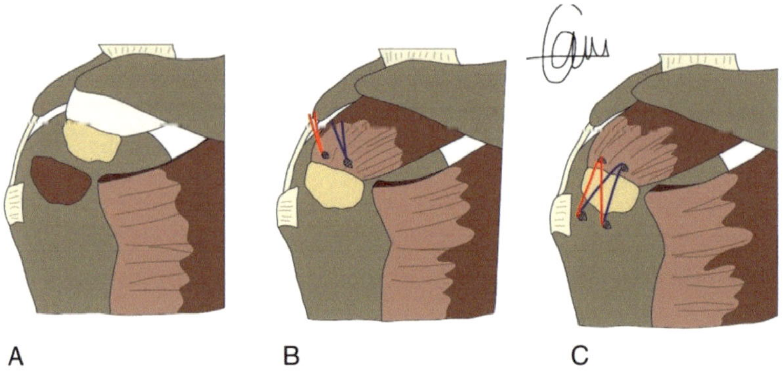

Figure 3.
Illustration of the arthroscopic reduction and double-row suture anchor fixation technique. A. GT fracture B. The 2 suture anchors are placed medial to the fracture bed, and the sutures are then threaded through the intact rotator cuff. C. Each of the two knotless anchors is loaded with a suture limb from each of the medial anchors before being inserted lateral to the fracture bed. The sutures are then tied above the fracture fragment to complete the repair.

important to use both views as relying on arthroscopic viewing without fluoroscopic viewing can lead to poor reduction.

We should remember that any concomitant pathology identified arthroscopically must be noted and repaired after fixing the fracture.

It is worth mentioning another arthroscopic technique widespread among the authors, which is the suture bridge technique with reported very good results and excellent satisfaction in practically all patients (**Figure 4**) [29–31].

Portals of entry, debridement of the fracture bed, and subsequent steps are common to the above-mentioned technique. The difference is that, here, we use different combinations of sutures. In this technique, we first insert two metal anchors at the articular margin of the humeral head through the intact cuff attached to the GT fragments [30]. A nylon is passed through a needle and then the four limbs of 1 double-loaded anchor are retrieved through the intact sleeve. The medial row sutures stitched over the fracture help to reduce it. With knotless anchors positioned in the vertical part of the tuberosity, distal to the fracture, sutures were tensioned and laterally secured. The lateral row anchors are inserted

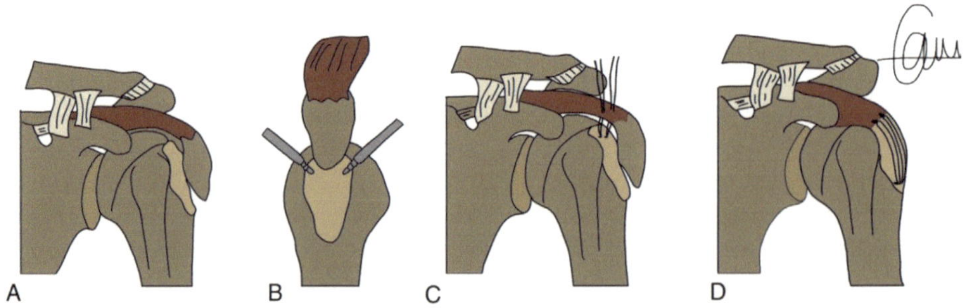

Figure 4.
Illustration of the arthroscopic suture bridge fixation technique. A. GT fracture; B. insert two metal anchors at the articular margin of the humeral head through the intact cuff attached to the GT fragments; C. A nylon is passed through a needle and then the four limbs of 1 double-loaded anchor are retrieved through the intact sleeve; D. Sutures are tensioned and secured over the fracture.

into the cortical bone of the proximal humerus. Due to the hardness of the cortical bone, it is recommended to pre-drill with the drill beat and then insert the lateral row anchors [29].

Another technique, the authors prefer, is the arthroscopic reduction and trans osseous augmented suture fixation technique useful in osteoporotic patients [32, 33]. A trans osseous tunnel is made, establishing the lateral entry point 2 cm below the lateral fracture margin to prevent cracking of the cortex. A lateral cortical augmentation can be used to avoid any peak stress on sound bone below the fracture margin [33]. An implant is then anchored with three different loaded sutures in the front eyelet of this implant. The sutures, exiting the trans osseous exit point toward the crater fracture, are passed posteriorly to the tendon of the avulsed fragment. Sutures are closed in a mattress fashion over the fragment reducing the fracture.

A parachute suture technique has been proposed for complicated fracture patterns, such as split, comminuted, or multi-fragmentary fracture patterns frequently treated with open reduction and internal fixation [34]. In this parachute arthroscopic procedure, four inverted horizontal knotless mattress sutures are combined with two reinforcing knotted mattress sutures for fracture fixation [35].

Among the different arthroscopic reduction alternatives, no clinical evidence exists that one is superior to the other. What has been shown is that suture anchor constructions may be superior in osteoporotic or multi-fragment fractures where plates or screws may further damage the fragments [28, 36].

3.3 Postoperative follow-up

Postoperative tuberosity fractures follow a protocol like the post-rotator cuff repair patient. Also, minimally displaced fractures of the greater tuberosity of the humerus can be associated with a rotator cuff tear, in this case, the prognosis is worse, and rehabilitation will have to be more focused on performing exercises to restore shoulder cinematics, with special focus in rotator cuff muscles [37].

In the immediate postoperative period of arthroscopic repair, the patient remains in an abduction sling to relieve tension on the supraspinatus tendon and greater tuberosity, one may support the arm in abduction, so the patient is placed in a sling with abduction. This can be done with an airplane splint or a shoulder abduction cushion. We need to focus on passive exercises while maintaining elbow and hand motion [36]. These passive exercises are initiated from the second postoperative day. Passive forward flexion and abduction are allowed and progressed gradually after 1 week preferably under physiotherapist supervision [36]. Formal physical therapy for active-assisted motion begins at 4 weeks, while strengthening exercises are initiated when radiographs showed apparent evidence of fracture healing, which commonly occurs 2–3 months after surgery.

Radiographs are regularly checked in the postoperative period to monitor fracture reduction and document healing [36]. At 6 weeks, active ROM exercises of the shoulder are usually performed and tolerated without pain.

After open reduction, patients are placed in a standard shoulder sling in the immediate postoperative period. The sling is worn for 4–6 weeks. Active motion of the elbow, wrist, and hand, as well as gentle passive exercises, are instituted since day one [20]. At 2 weeks, patients start formal, standardized physical therapy, including passive Range-of-motion (ROM) exercises for elevation and external rotation. At 6 weeks, they begin internal rotation stretching and active-assisted motion. Cuff strengthening begins gently, as motion and pain allowed, after 10–12 weeks. Formal physical therapy continues until full or maximal improvement in motion and strength has been achieved [18]. In general, the authors who applied open surgery started the exercises later than the groups that treat with arthroscopy.

However, some studies, such as that of Liao et al. [38], who compared open vs. arthroscopic surgery, described a similar rehabilitation protocol in the group treated with ORIF and the group treated with arthroscopy.

What is clear is that the literature tells us that the sooner rehabilitation is started in a safe and consensual manner, the better the results are in terms of mobility, stiffness, and residual pain. Even after significant reconstruction, early passive movement in accordance with pain tolerance can typically be started after the first postoperative day. The patient's capacity, expectations, and the strength and stability of the repair all need to be considered when designing the rehabilitation program.

3.4 Difference in outcomes between open and arthroscopic reduction

Huntley et al. [1] completed a systematic review that showed that patients treated arthroscopically reported slightly superior outcomes compared to patients receiving open reduction internal fixation. The open group had better postoperative forward flexion and external rotation, but the arthroscopic group had better abduction. But noted that most patients were satisfied with outcomes regardless of the technique used.

The extensive dissection required to expose the fracture fragments in open surgery can cause postoperative stiffness, and locking plates have been associated with a higher rate of subacromial impingement [38]. Irritation and protrusion of the hardware were frequently reported in the group treated with open surgery, which required reoperation; the arthroscopic reduction significantly reduced that complication [27]. As arthroscopic techniques improve, the indications for arthroscopic treatment of articular fractures expand. The main benefit of arthroscopic fixation of greater tuberosity fractures is that concurrent injuries, like labral and rotator cuff tears, can be identified and treated simultaneously [38].

The level of expertise required may constrain the use of arthroscopic repair in treating displaced greater tuberosity fractures. A properly executed open technique is preferable to a poorly executed arthroscopic procedure. Therefore, despite being an economically more expensive and technically demanding technique with a longer learning curve, arthroscopic reconstruction offers several advantages over open surgery that should not be ignored.

4. Non-surgical treatment

As we have mentioned, most authors recommend surgical treatment in active patients with a displacement greater than 5 mm and in athletes and workers involving force movements above the shoulder if the displacement is greater than 3 mm. In the literature, there are few examples of functional results in non-operatively treated patients with minimal displacement. Platzer et al. [10] studied displacements of the greater tuberosity of the humerus and the influence on the functionality of the humerus after recovery. Patients with a displacement between 1 and 3 mm and no displaced fractures had equal results. However, patients who had a displacement of more than 3 mm had worse outcomes than those with a smaller displacement, though this was statistically insignificant. Patients with a displacement of more than 5 mm did statistically worse. This supports the recommendation of surgical stabilization in athletes or heavy laborers with a displacement of more than 3 mm, and it should be considered in every active patient.

The period of immobilization varies from 1 to 4 weeks in studies [10, 39–42]. We discovered no significant differences in outcome even though Mitella slings were frequently used on younger patients and Gilchrist bandages were preferred for elderly patients to achieve immobilization [40]. After this period of immobilization, physiotherapy and rehabilitation programs with strengthening and mobility exercises are necessary.

Women and younger patients had significantly better results with non-operative treatments. Men showed a significant trend in secondary displacements [10].

Postoperative tuberosity fractures follow a protocol similar to the post-rotator cuff repair patient. Also, minimally displaced fractures of the greater tuberosity of the humerus can be associated with a rotator cuff tear; in this case, the prognosis is worse, and rehabilitation will have to be more focused on performing exercises to restore shoulder cinematics, with particular focus in rotator cuff muscles [37].

The patient is kept in an abduction sling for the first few days following surgery, focusing on passive exercises while maintaining elbow and hand motion [36]. On the second postoperative day, these pendulum exercises are begun. After a week, passive abduction and forward flexion are permitted and progress gradually [38]. Formal physical therapy for active-assisted motion starts at fourth week while strengthening exercises are initiated when radiographs show apparent evidence of fracture healing, commonly occurring 3 months after surgery.

Radiographs are regularly checked in the postoperative period to monitor fracture reduction and document healing [36]. At 6 weeks, active ROM exercises of the shoulder are usually performed and tolerated without pain.

5. Complications

A review was conducted in PubMed, Embase, and Scopus databases to identify relevant studies reporting complication rates in surgically managed greater tuberosity fractures [2, 43–52]. Outcomes were variable between series, with heterogeneous reports and data, and limited studies with high level of evidence were obtained. Complications were categorized into surgical site infection, nerve injury, implant-related issues, restricted range of motion, and other adverse events. The pooled complication rates for open and arthroscopic approaches were calculated based on each study's reported cases and total number of patients.

5.1 Open surgery complications

The pooled complication rate for open surgery was 17.2% (12.7–22.9%). Surgical site infections were the most common complication in 8.1% (4.7–13.9%) of cases. Nerve injuries were identified in 9.5% (5.8–15.4%) of patients. Implant-related complications were reported in 4.3% (2.1–8.5%) cases. Restricted range of motion and other complications collectively constituted 2.1% (0.9–4.9%) and 2.3% (1.0–5.3%) of cases, respectively.

5.2 Arthroscopic surgery complications

The pooled complication rate for arthroscopic surgery was 12.8% (8.3–19.5%). Notably, no surgical site infections were reported in the arthroscopic group. Nerve injuries were observed in 6.7% (4.0–11.1%) of patients. Implant-related complications occurred in 5.1% (2.7–9.5%) of cases. Restricted range of motion and other complications collectively constituted 1.9% (0.7–4.9%) and 1.7% (0.6–4.7%) of cases, respectively.

Based on the surgical approach, surgically treated greater tuberosity fractures exhibit varying complication rates. Arthroscopic techniques generally demonstrate lower overall complication rates, highlighting potential advantages such as reduced surgical site infections and comparable nerve injury rates.

Even we have found series with limited descriptions of shoulder stiffness, these complications have been described as the most frequent in proximal humeral surgery with rates as elevated as 25. To prevent it, formal physiotherapy is carried out with early and progressive passive range of motion and stretching [2]. The risks inherent to arthroscopic surgery must be considered, such as fluid extravasation, iatrogenic rotator cuff injury, cartilage injury, or neurovascular injury, especially the axillary nerve injury [27].

The neurological injuries frequently associated with fractures of the greater tuberosity of the humerus consist of injuries to the brachial plexus and the axillary nerve. In situations where there is a shoulder muscle weakness that is persistent, electromyography is very interesting. Less frequently occurring were vascular lesions (axillary artery and vein) [40].

6. Conclusion

Arthroscopic reduction and fixation of displaced GT fractures is a safe, effective, and minimally invasive procedure for optimal fracture healing and patient satisfaction and a reliable alternative to open fixation for fractures of the GT of the humerus.

We must emphasize the importance of having good preoperative images to not overlook concomitant injuries or secondary fracture patterns.

The arthroscopic technique has innumerable advantages, such as minimally invasive technique, allows you to visualize and addresses concomitant intraarticular pathology, some authors describe faster recovery [25], and no removal of implanted material when using the different suture systems. Other benefits of arthroscopic surgery include its minimally invasive nature, which results in less blood loss and soft tissue disruption, the ability to examine and treat other injured shoulder structures, reduced radiation exposure for both patient and doctor and improved biomechanical strength with suture anchor constructs [36].

On the other hand, the disadvantages of these techniques are that they are very technically challenging with an early learning curve, a longer operative time than open procedures, and visibility can be problematic in cases with significant bleeding. For this reason, they should be performed by expert shoulder surgeons with enough experience in arthroscopic procedures.

In most cases, greater tuberosity fractures can be successfully treated without surgery. However, patients with >5 mm superior GT displacement have better surgical treatment outcomes. Multiple surgical methods have been described for treating GT fractures and should be carefully and strategically employed according to comminution, displacement, type of patient, and morphology.

Conflict of interest

The authors declare no conflict of interest.

Author details

Raquel Guitián-Montes[1,2*], Samer Amhaz-Escanlar[3,4], Alberto Jorge-Mora[1,2,5] and Ana Carolina Presas-Presas[1]

1 Orthopaedic Department, Complejo Hospitalario de Pontevedra, Spain

2 TraumaSCQ, Santiago, Spain

3 Orthopaedic Department, Hospital Clínico Universitario de Santiago de Compostela, Spain

4 University of Santiago de Compostela, Spain

5 Musculoskeletal Pathology Group, Institute IDIS, Spain

*Address all correspondence to: publi.guitian@gmail.com

References

[1] Samuel R, Huntley A, Eva J, Lehtonen A, Joseph Xavier Robin A, Alexandra M, et al. Outcomes of surgical fixation of greater tuberosity fractures: A systematic review. Orthopaedics & Traumatology: Surgery & Research. 2020;**106**(6):1119-1126. DOI: 10.1016/j.otsr.2020.05.005

[2] Gruson KI, Ruchelsman DE, Tejwani NC. Isolated tuberosity fractures of the proximal humeral: Current concepts. Injury. 2008;**39**(3):284-298. DOI: 10.1016/j.injury.2007.09.022

[3] Rouleau DM, Mutch J, Laflamme GY. Surgical treatment of displaced greater tuberosity fractures of the humerus. The Journal of the American Academy of Orthopaedic Surgeons. 2016;**24**(1):46-56. DOI: 10.5435/JAAOS-D-14-00289

[4] Warner JJ, Costouros JG, Gerber C. Fractures of the proximal humerus. In: Bucholz RW, Heckman JD, Court-Brown C, editors. Rockwood & Green's Fractures in Adults. Ed. 6 ed. Philadelphia, PA: Lippincott William and Wilkins; 2006. pp. 1161-1209

[5] Le Minor JM, Tomasi JP, Segonds C, Duparc F. Arterial supply of the proximal humerus and its potential surgical applications. Surgical and Radiologic Anatomy. 2018;**40**(7):831-839

[6] Iacobellis C, Piccinini G, Sammartino A, Savarese E, Bisaccia M. Vascular anatomy of the greater and lesser tuberosities of the humerus: An angiographic study. Surgical and Radiologic Anatomy. 2019;**41**(6):663-667

[7] Basat HC, Aydin NK, Kizkapan TB, Yazicioglu O. Vascular anatomy of the humeral tuberosities and its relation to anatomical neck fractures: A cadaveric study. Journal of Orthopaedic Surgery and Research. 2017;**12**(1):40

[8] Standring S, Borley NR, Collins P, editors. Gray's Anatomy E-Book: The Anatomical Basis of Clinical Practice. Elsevier Health Sciences; 2016

[9] Hertel R, Hempfing A, Stiehler M, Leunig M. Predictors of humeral head ischemia after intracapsular fracture of the proximal humerus. Journal of Shoulder and Elbow Surgery. 2004;**13**(4):427-433. DOI: 10.1016/j.jse.2004.01.034

[10] Platzer P, Kutscha-Lissberg F, Lehr S, Vecsei V, Gaebler C. The influence of displacement on shoulder function in patients with minimally displaced fractures of the greater tuberosity. Injury. 2005;**36**(10):1185-1189

[11] White EA, Skalski MR, Patel DB, et al. Isolated greater tuberosity fractures of the proximal humerus: Anatomy, injury patterns, multimodality imaging, and approach to management. Emergency Radiology. 2018;**25**:235-246. DOI: 10.1007/s10140-018-1589-8

[12] Lorente A, Mariscal G, Barrios C, Lorente R. Nerve injuries after glenohumeral dislocation, a systematic review of incidence and risk factors. Journal of Clinical Medicine. 2023;**12**:4546. DOI: 10.3390/jcm12134546

[13] Patten RM, Mack LA, Wang KY, Lingel J. Nondisplaced fractures of the greater tuberosity of the humerus: Sonographic detection. Radiology. 1992;**182**:201-204

[14] Xue G, Chahal K, Lim T, Hu S, Li S, Liu J. Titanium mini locking plate with trans-osseous sutures for the

treatment of humeral greater tuberosity fracture osteosynthesis versus philos: A retrospective view. International Orthopaedics. 2018;**42**(10):2467-2473

[15] Gavaskar AS, Chowdary N, Abraham S. Complex proximal humerus fractures treated with locked plating utilizing an extended deltoid split approach with a shoulder strap incision. Journal of Orthopaedic Trauma. 2013;**27**(2):73-76. DOI: 10.1097/BOT.0b013e31825cf545

[16] Ju J, Ma M, Ding Z, Zhang Y. Clinical article. A transosseous suture as an alternative to suture anchor on anterior-avulsion greater tuberosity fragment fixation in neer three-part proximal humeral fracture: A biomechanical study. Orthopaedic Surgery. 2022;**15**(8):2132-2137

[17] Cheng MF, Hung SH, Su YP, Chiang CC, Chang MC, Chiu FY. Displaced isolated greater tuberosity fractures of elder adults treated with plate osteosynthesis. Journal of the Chinese Medical Association. 2019;**82**(4):318-321. DOI: 10.1097/JCMA.0000000000000049

[18] Gillespie RJ, Johnston PS, Gordon VA, Ward PJ, Getz CL. Using plate osteosynthesis to treat isolated greater tuberosity fractures. American Journal of Orthopedics (Belle Mead, N.J.). 2015;**44**(8):E248-E251

[19] Lee W, Shin H, Kim K. Open reduction and stable internal fixation using a 3.5-mm locking hook plate for isolated fractures of the greater tuberosity of the humerus: A 2-year follow-up study using an innovative fixation method. Clinics in Orthopedic Surgery. 2021;**13**:293-300

[20] Zeng LQ, Chen YF, Jiang YW, Zeng LL, Miao XG, Liang WG. A new low-profile anatomic locking plate for fixation of comminuted, displaced greater tuberosity fractures of the proximal humerus. Journal of Shoulder and Elbow Surgery. 2021;**30**(6):1402-1409. DOI: 10.1016/j.jse.2020.08.036 [Epub 2020 Sep 16]

[21] Xie L, Zhang Y, Chen C, Zheng W, Chen H, Cai L. Deltoid-split approach versus deltopectoral approach for proximal humerus fractures: A systematic review and meta-analysis. Orthopaedics & Traumatology, Surgery & Research. 2019;**105**(2):307-316. DOI: 10.1016/j.otsr.2018.12.004 [Epub 2019 Mar 14]

[22] Wu X, Li F, Ying J, Chen B, Su Y-X, Sun H-Y. Clinical effects between cannulated screw and bone plate internal fixation for humeral tuberosity fracture: A meta analysis. Zhongguo Gu Shang. 2021;**34**:180-190

[23] Liehu C, Weizong W, Shaojun S, Haihang L. Comparison of effectiveness between minimally invasive cannulated screw and open reduction and plate fixation in treatment of humeral greater tuberosity fracture. Chinese Journal of Reparative and Reconstructive Surgery. 2013;**27**(4):418-422

[24] Yoon T, Choi C, Choi Y. Clinical outcomes of minimally invasive open reduction and internal fixation by screw and washer for displaced greater tuberosity fracture of humerus. Journal of Shoulder and Elbow Surgery. 2017;**27**:1-5

[25] Godin JA, Katthagen JC, Fritz EM, Pogorzelski J, Millett PJ. Arthroscopic treatment of greater tuberosity avulsion fractures. Arthroscopy Techniques. 2017;**6**(3):e777-e783. DOI: 10.1016/j.eats.2017.02.006

[26] Ji JH, Shafi M, Song IS, Kim YY, McFarland EG, Moon CY. Arthroscopic

fixation technique for comminuted, displaced greater tuberosity fracture. Arthroscopy. 2010;**26**(5):600-609. DOI: 10.1016/j.arthro.2009.09.011 [Epub 2010 Feb 26]

[27] Kokkalis ZT, Papanikos E, Bavelou E, Togias G, Sioutis S, Mavrogenis AF, et al. Arthroscopic reduction and fixation of greater tuberosity fractures of the humerus. European Journal of Orthopaedic Surgery and Traumatology. 2021;**31**(6):1055-1060. DOI: 10.1007/s00590-020-02835-8 [Epub 2021 Jan 2]

[28] Patel SP, Nuelle CW, Hartzler RU. Arthroscopic reduction and internal fixation of proximal humerus greater tuberosity fracture. Arthroscopy Techniques. 2020;**9**(9):e1363-e1367. DOI: 10.1016/j.eats.2020.05.019

[29] Park SE, Ji JH, Shafi M, Jung JJ, Gil HJ, Lee HH. Arthroscopic management of occult greater tuberosity fracture of the shoulder. European Journal of Orthopaedic Surgery and Traumatology. 2014;**24**(4):475-482. DOI: 10.1007/s00590-013-1212-3 [Epub 2013 Apr 5]

[30] Ji JH, Jeong JJ, Kim YY, Lee SW, Kim DY, Park SE. Clinical and radiologic outcomes of arthroscopic suture bridge repair for the greater tuberosity fractures of the proximal humerus. Archives of Orthopaedic and Trauma Surgery. 2017;**137**(1):9-17. DOI: 10.1007/s00402-016-2586-6 [Epub 2016 Oct 26]

[31] Li R, Cai M, Tao K. Arthroscopic reduction and fixation for displaced greater tuberosity fractures using the modified suture-bridge technique. International Orthopaedics. 2017;**41**(6):1257-1263. DOI: 10.1007/s00264-017-3461-y [Epub 2017 Apr 11]

[32] Fleega BAN, Kareim S. Arthroscopic reduction and transosseous suture fixation of avulsed displaced shoulder greater tuberosity fracture. Arthroscopy Techniques. 2021;**10**(3):e821-e830. DOI: 10.1016/j.eats.2020.10.074

[33] Chillemi C, Proietti R, Rengo M, Damo M, Paolicelli D, Castagna A. Fracture avulsion of the greater tuberosity: Arthroscopic transosseous augmented technique. Arthroscopy Techniques. 2021;**10**(5):e1233-e1238. DOI: 10.1016/j.eats.2021.01.017

[34] Velasquez Garcia A, Abdo G, Ingala ML. Arthroscopic parachute technique for split-type greater tuberosity fractures. Arthroscopy Techniques. 2023;**12**(3):e349-e355. DOI: 10.1016/j.eats.2022.11.014

[35] Stueve J, Fenlin J. The parachute technique: Repair of displaced 2-part proximal humerus fractures. Techniques in Shoulder & Elbow Surgery. 2009;**10**:125-129. DOI: 10.1097/BTE.0b013e3181b3555c

[36] Andrew H, Larry F. Arthroscopic management of displaced greater tuberosity fractures. Arthroscopy Techniques. 2021;**10**:e1055-e1060. DOI: 10.1016/j.eats.2020.12.006

[37] Fjalestad T, Hole MØ, Blücher J, Hovden IA, Stiris MG, Strømsøe K. Rotator cuff tears in proximal humeral fractures: An MRI cohort study in 76 patients. Archives of Orthopaedic and Trauma Surgery. 2010;**130**(5):575-581. DOI: 10.1007/s00402-009-0953-2 [Epub 2009 Aug 14]

[38] Liao W, Zhang H, Li Z, Li J. Is arthroscopic technique superior to open reduction internal fixation in the treatment of isolated displaced greater tuberosity fractures? Clinical Orthopaedics and Related Research. 2016;**474**(5):1269-1279. DOI: 10.1007/s11999-015-4663-5 [Epub 2016 Jan 4]

[39] Kumar S, Mishra A, Singh H, Clark D, Espag M, Tambe A. Surgical fixation of isolated greater tuberosity fractures of the humerus-systematic review and meta-analysis. Journal of Clinical Orthopaedics and Trauma. 2021;**23**:101670. DOI: 10.1016/j.jcot.2021.101670

[40] Jellad A, Bouaziz MA, Boudokhane S, Aloui I, Ben Salah Z, Abid A. Isolated greater tuberosity fracture: Short-term functional outcome following a specific rehabilitation program. Annals of Physical and Rehabilitation Medicine. 2012;**55**(1):16-24. English, French. Epub 2011 Dec 3. DOI: 10.1016/j.rehab.2011.10.007

[41] Mattyasovszky SG, Burkhart KJ, Ahlers C, Proschek D, Dietz SO, Becker I, et al. Isolated fractures of the greater tuberosity of the proximal humerus: A long-term retrospective study of 30 patients. Acta Orthopaedica. 2011;**82**(6):714-720. DOI: 10.3109/17453674.2011.618912 [Epub 2011 Sep 6]

[42] Rath E, Alkrinawi N, Levy O, Debbi R, Amar E, Atoun E. Minimally displaced fractures of the greater tuberosity: Outcome of non-operative treatment. Journal of Shoulder and Elbow Surgery. 2013;**22**(10):e8-e11. DOI: 10.1016/j.jse.2013.01.033 [Epub 2013 Apr 29]

[43] Torrens C, Alentorn-Geli E, Mingo F, Gamba C, Santana F. Reverse shoulder arthroplasty for the treatment of acute complex proximal humeral fractures: Influence of greater tuberosity healing on the functional outcomes. Journal of Orthopaedic Surgery (Hong Kong). Jan-Apr 2018;**26**(1):2309499018760132. DOI: 10.1177/2309499018760132. PMID: 29486672

[44] Verdano MA, Aliani D, Pellegrini A, Baudi P, Pedrazzi G, Cec-carelli F. Isolated fractures of the greater tuberosity in proximal humerus: Does the direction of displacement influence functional outcome? An analysis of displacement in greater tuberosity fractures. Acta Biomedica. 2013;**84**(3):219-228

[45] Yin B, Moen TC, Thompson SA, Bigliani LU, Ahmad CS, Levine WN. Operative treatment of isolated greater tuberosity fractures: Retrospective review of clinical and functional outcomes. Orthopedics. 2012;**35**(6):e807-e814

[46] Platzer P, Thalhammer G, Oberleitner G, et al. Displaced fractures of the greater tuberosity: A comparison of operative and nonoperative treatment. Journal of Trauma and Acute Care Surgery. 2008;**65**(4):843-848

[47] McLaughlin HL. Dislocation of the shoulder with tuberosity fracture. Surgical Clinics of North America. 1963;**43**:1615-1620

[48] Dimakopoulos P, Panagopoulos A, Kasimatis G, Syggelos SA, Lambiris E. Anterior traumatic shoulder dislocation associated with displaced greater tuberosity fracture: The necessity of operative treatment. Journal of Orthopaedic Trauma. 2007;**21**(2):104-112

[49] Chen CY, Chao EK, Tu YK, Ueng SW, Shih CH. Closed management and percutaneous fixation of unstable proximal humerus fractures. Journal of Trauma and Acute Care Surgery. 1998;**45**(6):1039-1045

[50] Ji JH, Shafi M, Song IS, Kim YY, McFarland EG, Moon CY. Arthroscopic fixation technique for comminuted, displaced greater tuberosity fracture. Arthroscopy: The Journal of Arthroscopic & Related Surgery. 2010;**26**(5):600-609

[51] Bhatia DN, van Rooyen KS, Toit du DF, de Beer JF. Surgical treatment of comminuted, displaced fractures of the greater tuberosity of the proximal humerus: A new technique of double-row suture-anchor fixation and long-term results. Injury. 2006;**37**(10):946-952

[52] Rojas JT, Rashid MS, Zumstein MA. How to treat stiffness after proximal humeral fractures? EFORT Open Reviews. 1 Aug 2023;**8**(8):651-661. DOI: 10.1530/EOR-22-0118. PMID: 37526247; PMCID: PMC10441249

Chapter 4

Arthroscopic Tenotomy versus Open Tenodesis of the Long Head Biceps Brachii Tendon

Matilde Delvecchio, Gian Mario Micheloni, Andrea Giorgini and Giuseppe Porcellini

Abstract

The aim of the chapter is to compare the surgical treatment of tendinopathies of the long head of the biceps brachii, in particular arthroscopic tenotomy versus open tenodesis. Arthroscopic tenotomy of the long head of the biceps tendon is the preferred technique in cases where pain is to be relieved and in cases where the long head is subluxated with injury to the upper fibers of the subscapularis muscle. Subpectoral open tenodesis of the long head of the biceps tendon may be the preferable technique in selected cases of younger patients, athletes, or with high functional demand; in these cases, a good recovery of muscle strength, less muscle cramping, and less imperfection should be achieved.

Keywords: tenodesis, tenotomy, long head biceps brachii, arthroscopy, shoulder pain

1. Introduction

The pathology of the long head of the biceps brachii (LHB) tendon can cause shoulder pain, in particular anterior shoulder pain. Although it may also manifest as a primary isolated LHB tendinopathy, this condition is frequently linked to rotator cuff tendinopathy.

The LHB's functional role has been and continues to be poorly understood.

According to several experimental and clinical research, the LHB tendon may function as a glenoid labrum elevator, an anterior stabilizer, a posterior stabilizer, and a depressor of the humeral head [1–3].

Following tenotomy or tenodesis, these functions might disappear.

LHB tendon pathology can be classified into three different categories: LHB degeneration (peritendinous, inflammation, hypertrophy, partial or complete tear), LHB anchor disorders (SLAP lesions), and LH instability (subluxation or dislocation) [4].

Regarding the surgical management of LHB tendinopathy, there is still no universal agreement: some support tenotomy while others support tenodesis.

Tenotomy is a simple surgical technique that can be carried out using an arthroscopic procedure. A postoperative Popeye deformity in the upper arm that is accompanied by pain and/or cramping in the retracted muscle can be linked to this operation.

Technically more difficult and need a longer duration of recuperation is LHB tenodesis. The tenodesis of the biceps brachii is said to increase strength, however, this is not well supported in the literature.

2. Long head biceps brachii tendon

2.1 Anatomy of LHBT

The long head biceps tendon is a structure of the glenohumeral joint. It originates from the supraglenoid tubercle and glenoid superior labrum, with the proximal tendon moving laterally into the rotator cuff interval before being encircled by the biceps pulley and housed in the biceps groove. A common distal tendon attachment onto the radial tuberosity ligament is shared by the muscle when it leaves the biceps pulley and passes underneath the transverse humeral ligament to form the biceps brachii muscle belly [5].

2.2 Anatomical variations

Anatomical variations are very common. The most common observed anatomical variations included aberrant origins, supernumerary accessory heads and LHBT absence [6, 7]. The most common aberrant origin of the LHB at the shoulder is the presence of a bifurcate tendon origin and an anomalous LHBT origin from the supraspinatus [8]. In rare cases, there may be a trifurcated origin or four-headed biceps variant. In some shoulders, no anatomic structure distinct from the transverse humeral ligament can be recognized to support a role in the stability of the LHBT in the bicipital groove [9].

A positive correlation was found between observed anatomical variances of the LHBT origin and the presence of anterosuperior labral fraying, abnormal superior glenohumeral ligament [7], and LHBT absence and the presence of shoulder pain and instability [10].

2.3 Function of LHBT

The functional role of LHBT at the shoulder and its contribution to glenohumeral joint biomechanics and stability is not clearly understood [11]. Some researchers think that LHBT has a role in humeral head depression and stabilization, whereas some others suggest that the tendon plays no role [12]. A considerable superior migration of the head of the humerus was observed after tenotomy in a large study of 291 patients undergoing LHB tenotomy for irreparable full-thickness rips of the rotator cuff, by Walch and Edwards [13].

2.4 Lesions

LHB tendon pathology can be classified into three different categories: LHB degeneration (peritendinous, inflammation, hypertrophy, partial or complete tear), LHB anchor disorders (SLAP lesions), and LH instability (subluxation or dislocation) [4, 14].

These are common cause of anterior shoulder pain with associated dysfunction of forward flexion and disorders in patients with rotator cuff tears [15].

2.5 Clinical examination

Clinical examination can be conducted with objective examination, instrumental investigations, such as ultrasonography and MRI.

When conducting a clinical study, it is important to investigate symptoms like pain, evaluate stability, and check for any structural abnormalities.

One of the most important diagnostic criteria has been a precise patient history that includes a description of the mechanism of injury.

It is possible to look for Popeye's sign, a bulge on the medial side of the upper arm that becomes more noticeable with vigorous or resistant elbow flexion and has a different aspect from the opposite arm was described as Popeye sign.

According to research, the LHB is innervated by a network of sensory sympathetic fibers, particularly near its beginning, which may contribute to the pathogenesis of shoulder discomfort [16].

LHB pathologic physical examination is difficult, because at the time of testing, cartilage disease and typically concurrent soft tissue pathology (rotator cuff, pulleys, labrum) interfere. Additionally, there is no recognized pain pattern unique to the biceps tendon.

Clinical objectivity is studied by some clinical tests, such as biceps groove palpation, Speed's, Yergason's, and Uppercut test.

Speed's test: the patient is asked to flex the arm against resistance while keeping the elbow extended and the forearm supinated; the test is positive if there is pain at the biceps groove; Holtby reports a sensitivity of 32% and a specificity of 75% [17].

Yergason's test: the patient flexes the elbow to 90° while keeping the arm adducted to the chest, then asked to supinate the forearm against resistance; in case of pain at the bicipital groove, the test is positive; Holtby reports a sensitivity of 43% and specificity of 79% [17, 18].

Uppercut test: the patient is posed with the shoulder in neutral rotation and the elbow flexed to 90°, the forearm is supinated and the patient clenches his fingers into a fist, then the examiner grasps the patient's fist and invites the patient to make a movement against resistance similar to an uppercut; the test is positive in case of anterior pain [17, 19].

Arthroscopy is by far the most accurate diagnostic investigation of proximal biceps pathology.

The Constant score is still utilized in most studies as the primary outcome score after rotator cuff surgery since biceps therapy is still considered to be an important component of treatment and the long biceps tendon is located proximal to the supraspinatus tendon, which is typically affected [20].

2.6 Treatment

In most cases, conservative management is preferred, which includes rest, nonsteroidal anti-inflammatory medicines, physical therapy, and steroid injections.

Surgery is frequently recommended if symptoms that have been treated conservatively for more than 3 months continue [21].

Surgical treatment of LHB tendon is also recommended in cases of isolated symptomatic pathology, such as SLAP II (or higher stages of Snyder classification), partial tears, hour-glass deformity, or in concomitant rotator cuff lesions with biceps instability and tendinitis and finally at the time of shoulder arthroplasty [22].

Both open and arthroscopic procedures are part of the surgical strategy. An increasing number of surgeons now advocate arthroscopic management [23].

2.6.1 Tenotomy

Depending on the surgeon's preference, shoulder arthroscopy is performed while the patient is in the lateral decubitus or beach chair position.

Diagnostic arthroscopy is performed with a standard posterior portal and a standard anterior interval portal is used to evaluate the biceps tendon, using an arthroscopic probe. The identification of ripping, instability, degeneration, or inflammation of the long head of the biceps tendon or superior labrum attachment is used to confirm the study's final eligibility. For patients who had a biceps tenotomy, the surgeon used an arthroscopic biter, an electrothermal device, or a knife to separate the long head of the biceps tendon from its proximal anchor to the superior labrum [24].

Tenotomy is a surgical procedure that might involve either releasing the LHB with a portion of superior labrum or just cutting the tendon at the very base of the origin. The final alternative, known as the "fish tail" or "T-wedge" approach, catches beneath the transverse humeral ligament and is occasionally recognized as a soft tissue tenodesis [22]. Tenotomy is much easier to perform and requires less complicated rehabilitation, and it allows an earlier return to daily activities [25].

2.6.2 Tenodesis

Tenodesis is performed by arthroscopic, open, or mini-open surgery. It can also be separated into fixation methods for soft tissue, osseous, and intraosseous structures, with or without the use of implants [22]. The approach used for LHB tenodesis may occasionally be determined by concurrent disease, such as rotator cuff or labral pathology, but the treating surgeon ultimately has the final say.

Open vs. arthroscopic approaches, fixation methods, and tenodesis locations—generally referred to as suprapectoral or subpectoral—are all technical issues. The level may be distal subpectoral, suprapectoral, intra-articular, or proximal intra-articular. It is crucial to preserve the link between muscle length and tension and avoid overtightening the final fixation [22].

Open LHB tenodesis is usually performed subpectorally. Initially, a biceps tenotomy is performed at the biceps-labral junction with an arthroscopic scissor or basket; then an axillary incision of about 3 cm centered on the lower edge of the pectoralis major is made; the arm is intrarotolated, and the lower edge of the pectoralis major is retracted bluntly upward to allow probing of the biceps groove and biceps tendon. Following the release of the tendon, the proximal tendon is removed and a braided suture 15 mm proximal to the myotendinous junction is performed and a bioabsorbable interference screw connected to the pectoralis major tendon is inserted until the screw rests against the anterior cortical surface of the humerus. Finally, the ends of the suture are tied and cut to secure it [26].

Tenodesis can also be performed *via* suprapectoral arthroscopy. The biceps tendon is marked with a suture, then a biceps tenotomy is performed at the level of the biceps-labral junction. A subacromial bursectomy is performed to visualize the ligaments covering the tendon in the groove. The biceps tendon is electrocauterized, and the marked portion of the tendon is then extracted from the anterolateral portal. The proximal 15 mm of the tendon is removed and replaced with a braided locking suture. A bone tunnel is then performed on a guide wire inserted in the bicipital groove and a bioabsorbable tenodesis is performed to fix the tendon to the proximal humerus [26].

Subacromial decompression is performed with a cutting block technique if required, and the rotator cuff is repaired if necessary, *via* standard antero- and posterolateral accessory portals based on tear configuration [24].

The success of the therapy as a whole, as determined by patient-reported outcomes, should not be primarily attributed to the tenodesis procedure itself, as LHB tenodesis is frequently carried out in conjunction with other procedures, it should be noted [26].

3. Arthroscopic tenotomy versus open tenodesis of the long head biceps brachii tendon

Although both tenotomy and tenodesis can benefit LHBT lesions, no consensus has been formed about which procedure is better. In numerous research [23, 27–29] the effectiveness of biceps tenotomy and various tenodesis procedures in the treatment of LHB lesions has been compared; nevertheless, the best surgical plan is still up for debate. Although it does not improve shoulder strength, biceps tenotomy or tenodesis reduces pain and improves the functional range of motion (**Figures 1–3**) [28].

The simple and well-tolerated arthroscopic biceps tenotomy method reduces operating time, streamlines postoperative rehabilitation, and enables patients to resume normal activities as soon as feasible [30].

However, there are certain disadvantages to the treatment, such as the potential deformity of the arm's anatomic profile (Popeye sign), the possibility of cramping and fatigue pain, and biomechanical modifications to the humeral head's response to LHBT capacity [10].

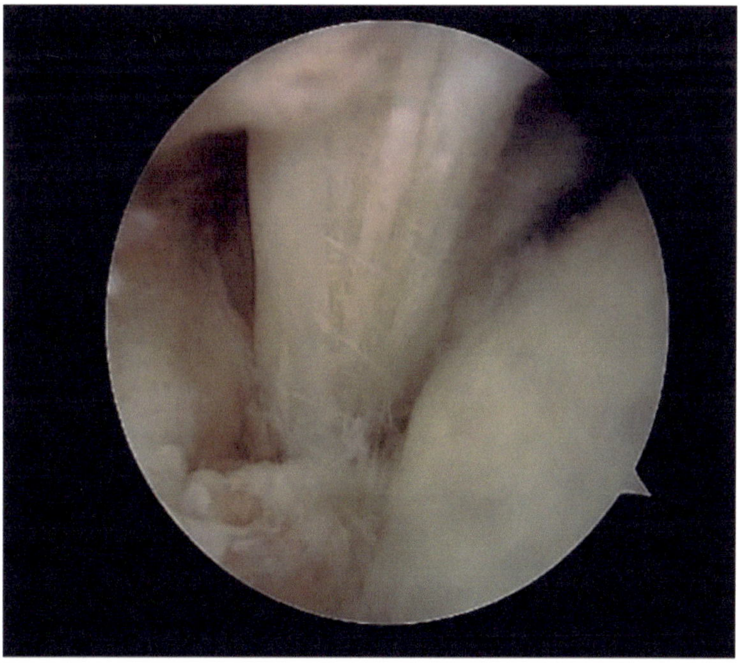

Figure 1.
Lesion of LHBT.

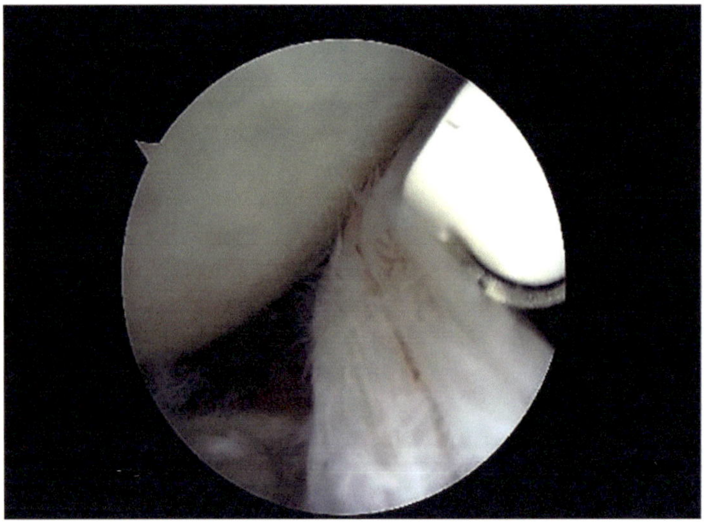

Figure 2.
Arthroscopic stability test.

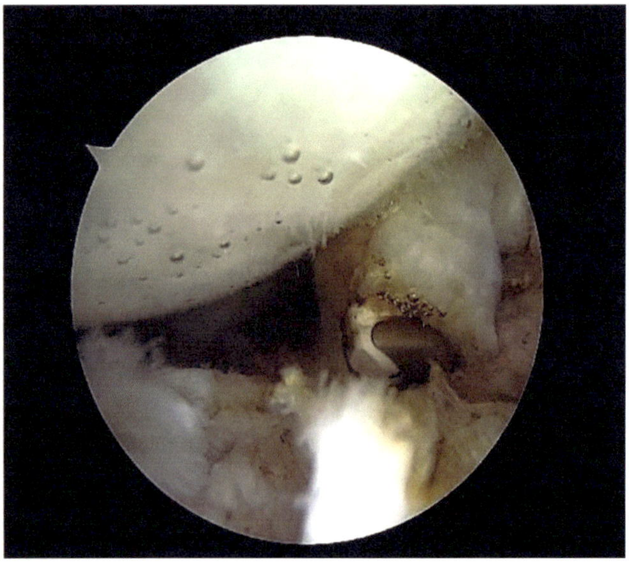

Figure 3.
Arthroscopic tenotomy of LHBT.

Tenotomy and tenodesis have different rates of esthetic deformity (Popeye sign) at 43 and 8%, respectively [21].

However, while LHB tenotomy was more frequently linked to a Popeye deformity, Gurnani et al. did discover a difference in the upper arm's esthetic look and cramping pain: following every LHB tendon tenotomy and tenodesis, the Popeye deformity was not present [20]. These findings may be explained by auto-tenodesis of the LHB, following tenotomy in the bicipital groove and failure of the tenodesis [31]. Inflammation in the bicipital groove or rotator interval may stimulate the biceps tendon to undergo autotenodesis and the time of immobilization after rotator cuff surgery may also affect the autotenodesis, resulting in less Popeye abnormalities [14].

Tenotomy is surgically simpler to do than tenodesis since no fixation is necessary, but it is more likely to cause muscle cramping, the Popeye sign, decreased elbow flexion, and decreased supination power [14, 25, 32, 33]. One of the main reason for preferred tenotomy is simplicity [31]. Tenotomy requires less rehabilitation and immobilization, yields better functional outcomes, and enables an earlier resumption of daily activities [27].

Tenotomy is a very straightforward and repeatable operation that greatly reduces shoulder discomfort without the need for postoperative rehabilitation [14]. Compared to tenodesis, arthroscopic tenotomy achieves comparable levels of postoperative discomfort and patient satisfaction [12].

Pain at the bicipital groove may be greater for those undergoing a subpectoral biceps tenodesis [34], however, biceps tenotomy is associated with earlier pain relief after surgical treatment of LHB tendinopathy [35].

Tenotomy is therefore often recommended for older, inactive individuals who are less concerned with the esthetic outcome, and who are not engaged in physically demanding or heavy labor tasks [36].

Due to the drawbacks of tenotomy, some surgeons support tenodesis, which, despite longer recovery periods and a more technically challenging procedure, results in a better ability to return to activity, a lower incidence of cosmetic deformities and cramping pain, and a closer approximation of normal anatomy [10].

Treatment algorithms generally recommend tenodesis for younger patients or those with cosmetic concerns.

Both procedures produce great therapeutic results, however, younger people, athletes, and patients who are concerned about their appearance cosmetically should consider tenodesis. By maintaining the LHBT length-tension relationship, it enables a better recovery to physical activity while being a longer and more expensive treatment that also necessitates longer rehabilitation [37].

The scar cosmesis may also play a role in patients' assent since biceps tenodesis frequently replaces tenotomy due to its enhanced cosmetic appearance [36].

Tenodesis seem to have superior forearm supination strength and Constant scores and to have a less rate of "Popeye" deformity than tenotomy [38].

Tenodesis, despite requiring more technical skill and a longer period of postoperative rehabilitation, it offers a quicker return to physical activity, less cosmetic abnormalities, and a better alignment with normal anatomy [37].

Concerns have been raised that using the open technique could increase the risk of wound complications and nerve damage [39].

While patient opinion of open tenodesis compared to arthroscopic tenodesis has not been examined, it can be a significant factor in selecting surgical treatment together with surgeon experience and choice.

In conclusion, the surgical prephgfference and technical experience of the surgeons should be taken into consideration when deciding whether to execute the tenodesis using an open or arthroscopic method.

Conflict of interest

The authors declare no conflict of interest.

Author details

Matilde Delvecchio*, Gian Mario Micheloni, Andrea Giorgini and Giuseppe Porcellini
Orthopedic and Traumatology Department, University of Modena and Reggio Emilia, Modena, Italy

*Address all correspondence to: matilde.delvecchio95@gmail.com

References

[1] Gill TJ, McIrvin E, Mair SD, Hawkins RJ. Results of biceps tenotomy for treatment of pathology of the long head of the biceps brachii. Journal of Shoulder and Elbow Surgery. 2001;**10**(3):247-249

[2] Levy AS, Kelly BT, Lintner SA, Osbahr DC, Speer KP. Function of the long head of the biceps at the shoulder: Electromyographic analysis. Journal of Shoulder and Elbow Surgery. 2001;**10**(3):250-255

[3] Rodosky MW, Harner CD, Fu FH. The role of the long head of the biceps muscle and superior glenoid labrum in anterior stability of the shoulder. The American Journal of Sports Medicine. 1994;**22**(1):121-130

[4] Scheibel M, Schröder RJ, Chen J, Bartsch M. Arthroscopic soft tissue tenodesis versus bony fixation anchor tenodesis of the long head of the biceps tendon. The American Journal of Sports Medicine. 2011;**39**(5):1046-1052

[5] Gray H, Williams PL, Bannister LH. Gray's anatomy: The anatomical basis of medicine and surgery. In: Bannister LH et al., editors. 38th/Chairman of the Editorial Board, Peter L. Williams; Editorial Board. New York: Churchill Livingstone; 1995

[6] Kosugi K, Shibata S, Yamashita H. Supernumerary head of biceps brachii and 51. Branching pattern of the musculocutaneus nerve in Japanese. Surgical and Radiologic Anatomy. 1992;**14**(2):175-185

[7] Rao AG, Kim TK, Chronopoulos E, McFarland EG. Anatomical variants in the anterosuperior aspect of the glenoid Labrum. The Journal of Bone and Joint Surgery. 2003;**85**(4):653

[8] Enad JG. Bifurcate origin of the long head of the biceps tendon. Arthroscopy. 2004;**20**(10):1081-1083

[9] Diplock B, Hing W, Marks D. The long head of biceps at the shoulder: A scoping review. BMC Musculoskeletal Disorders. 2023;**24**(1):232. DOI: 10.1186/s12891-023-06346-5

[10] Kumar CD, Rakesh J, Tungish B, Singh DM. Congenital absence of the long head of biceps tendon and its clinical implications: A systematic review of the literature. Muscles Ligaments & Tendons Journal (MLTJ). 2017;7(3):562-569

[11] Elser F, Braun S, Dewing CB, Giphart JE, Millett PJ. Anatomy, function, injuries, and treatment of the long head of the biceps brachii tendon. Arthroscopy. 2011;**27**(4):581-592

[12] Ge H, Zhang Q, Sun Y, Li J, Sun L, Cheng B. Tenotomy or tenodesis for the long head of biceps lesions in shoulders: A systematic review and meta-analysis. PLoS One. 2015;**10**(3):e0121286. DOI: 10.1371/journal.pone.0121286

[13] Walch G, Edwards TB, Boulahia A, Nové-Josserand L, Neyton L, Szabo I. Arthroscopic tenotomy of the long head of the biceps in the treatment of rotator cuff tears: Clinical and radiographic results of 307 cases. J Shoulder Elbow Surg. May-Jun 2005;**14**(3):238-246. DOI: 10.1016/j.jse.2004.07.008. PMID: 15889020

[14] Koh KH, Ahn JH, Kim SM, Yoo JC. Treatment of biceps tendon lesions in the setting of rotator cuff tears: Prospective cohort study of tenotomy versus tenodesis. The American Journal of Sports Medicine. 2010;**38**:1584-1590. DOI: 10.1177/0363546510364053

[15] Na Y, Zhu Y, Shi Y, Ren Y, Zhang T, Liu W, et al. A meta-analysis comparing tenotomy or tenodesis for lesions of the long head of the biceps tendon with concomitant reparable rotator cuff tears. Journal of Orthopaedic Surgery and Research. 2019;**14**(1):370. DOI: 10.1186/s13018-019-1429-x

[16] Alpantaki K, McLaughlin D, Karagogeos D, Hadjipavlou A, Kontakis G. Sympathetic and sensory neural elements in the tendon of the long head of the biceps. The Journal of Bone and Joint Surgery. American Volume. 2005;**87-A**:1580-1583

[17] Holtby R, Razmjou H. Accuracy of the Speed's and Yergason's tests in detecting biceps pathology and SLAP lesions: Comparison with arthroscopic findings. Arthroscopy. 2004;**20**(3):231-236. DOI: 10.1016/j.arthro.2004.01.008

[18] Yergason RM. Supination sign. Journal of Bone and Joint Surgery. 1931;**131**:160

[19] Ben Kibler W, Sciascia AD, Hester P, Dome D, Jacobs C. Clinical utility of traditional and new tests in the diagnosis of biceps tendon injuries and superior labrum anterior and posterior lesions in the shoulder. The American Journal of Sports Medicine. 2009;**37**(9):1840-1847. DOI: 10.1177/0363546509332505 Epub 2009 Jun 9

[20] Gurnani N, van Deurzen DF, Janmaat VT, van den Bekerom MP. Tenotomy or tenodesis for pathology of the long head of the biceps brachii: A systematic review and meta-analysis. Knee Surgery, Sports Traumatology, Arthroscopy. 2016;**24**(12):3765-3771. DOI: 10.1007/s00167-015-3640-6 Epub 2015 May 15

[21] Slenker NR, Lawson K, Ciccotti MG, Dodson CC, Cohen SB. Biceps tenotomy versus tenodesis: Clinical outcomes. Arthroscopy. 2012;**28**:576-582. DOI: 10.1016/j.arthro.2011.10.017

[22] Arthroscopy Basic to Advanced. Randelli. Dejour, Seil, Dijk: Denti; 2016

[23] Cho NS, Cha SW, Rhee YG. Funnel tenotomy versus intracuff tenodesis for lesions of the long head of the biceps tendon associated with rotator cuff tears. The American Journal of Sports Medicine. 2014;**42**:1161-1168. DOI: 10.1177/0363546514523719

[24] MacDonald P, Verhulst F, McRae S, Old J, Stranges G, Dubberley J, et al. Biceps Tenodesis versus Tenotomy in the treatment of lesions of the long head of the biceps tendon in patients undergoing arthroscopic shoulder surgery: A prospective double-blinded randomized controlled trial. The American Journal of Sports Medicine. 2020;**48**(6):1439-1449. DOI: 10.1177/0363546520912212 Epub 2020 Mar 30

[25] Wittstein JR, Queen R, Abbey A, Toth A, Moorman CT III. Isokinetic strength, endurance, and subjective outcomes after biceps tenotomy versus tenodesis. The American Journal of Sports Medicine. 2011;**39**:857-865

[26] Duchman KR, DeMik DE, Uribe B, Wolf BR, Bollier M. Open versus arthroscopic biceps Tenodesis: A comparison of functional outcomes. The Iowa Orthopaedic Journal. 2016;**36**:79-87

[27] Franceschi F, Longo UG, Ruzzini L, Rizzello G, Maffulli N, et al. No advantages in repairing a type II superior labrum anterior and posterior (SLAP) lesion when associated with rotator cuff repair in patients over age 50: A randomized controlled trial. The American Journal of Sports Medicine. 2008;**36**:247-253

[28] Boileau P, Baque F, Valerio L, Ahrens P, Chuinard C, et al. Isolated

arthroscopic biceps tenotomy or tenodesis improves symptoms in patients with massive irreparable rotator cuff tears. The Journal of Bone and Joint Surgery. American Volume. 2007;**89**:747-757

[29] Zhang Q, Zhou J, Ge H, Cheng B. Tenotomy or tenodesis for long head biceps lesions in shoulders with reparable rotator cuff tears: A prospective randomised trial. Knee Surgery, Sports Traumatology, Arthroscopy. 2015;**23**(2):464-469. DOI: 10.1007/s00167-013-2587-8 Epub 2013 Jul 5

[30] Kelly AM, Drakos MC, Fealy S, Taylor SA, O'Brien SJ. Arthroscopic release of the long head of the biceps tendon: Functional outcome and clinical results. The American Journal of Sports Medicine. 2005;**33**:208-213

[31] Frost A, Zafar MS, Maffulli N. Tenotomy versus tenodesis in the management of pathologic lesions of the tendon of the long head of the biceps brachii. The American Journal of Sports Medicine. 2009;**37**(4):828-833

[32] Oh JH, Lee YH, Kim SH, Park JS, Seo HJ, Kim W, et al. Comparison of treatments for superior labrum–biceps complex lesions with concomitant rotator cuff repair: A prospective, randomized, comparative analysis of debridement, biceps tenotomy, and biceps tenodesis. Arthroscopy. 2016;**32**(6):958-967 Epub 2016 Feb 23

[33] Shank JR, Singleton SB, Braun S, Kissenberth MJ, Ramappa A, Ellis H, et al. A comparison of forearm supination and elbow flexion strength in patients with long head of the biceps tenotomy or tenodesis. Arthroscopy. 2011;**27**(1):9-16 Epub 2010 Oct 29

[34] Friedman JL, FitzPatrick JL, Rylander LS, Bennett C, Vidal AF, McCarty EC. Biceps Tenotomy versus Tenodesis in active patients younger than 55 years: Is there a difference in strength and outcomes? Orthopaedic Journal of Sports Medicine. 2015;**3**(2):2325967115570848. DOI: 10.1177/2325967115570848

[35] Belay ES, Wittstein JR, Garrigues GE, Lassiter TE, Scribani M, Goldner RD, et al. Biceps tenotomy has earlier pain relief compared to biceps tenodesis: A randomized prospective study. Knee Surgery, Sports Traumatology, Arthroscopy. 2019;**27**(12):4032-4037. DOI: 10.1007/s00167-019-05682-1 Epub 2019 Sep 5

[36] Galdi B, Southren DL, Brabston EW, Popkin CA, Jobin CM, Levine WN, et al. Patients have strong preferences and perceptions for biceps tenotomy versus tenodesis. Arthroscopy. 2016;**32**(12):2444-2450 Epub 2016 Jun 16

[37] Werner BC, Lyons ML, Evans CL, Griffin JW, Hart JM, Miller MD, et al. Arthroscopic suprapectoral and open subpectoral biceps tenodesis: A comparison of restoration of length-tension and mechanical strength between techniques. Arthroscopy. 2015;**31**(4):620-627 Epub 2014 Dec 10

[38] Hartland AW, Islam R, Teoh KH, Rashid MS. Clinical effectiveness of tenotomy versus tenodesis for long head of biceps pathology: A systematic review and meta-analysis. BMJ Open. 2022;**12**(10):e061954. DOI: 10.1136/bmjopen-2022-061954

[39] Jeong HY, Kim JY, Cho NS, Rhee YG. Biceps lesion associated with rotator cuff tears: Open subpectoral and arthroscopic intracuff tenodesis. Orthopaedic Journal of Sports Medicine. 2016;**4**(5):2325967116645311

Chapter 5

Assessment of Upper Trapezium Pain and Muscle Strength after Posiconal Release and Myofascial Release

Allyson Cabral and Paulo Veiga

Abstract

Myofascial Pain Syndrome is characterized by sensory, motor, and autonomic symptoms caused by myofascial trigger points (TPs), resulting in quality of life, daily and social activities. The objective is to compare the levels of strength and pain tolerance before and after the use of Positional Release (TLP) and Myofascial Release (TLM) techniques. This is carried out as cross-sectional, quantitative, experimental study. Individuals with myofascial trigger points in the upper trapezius participated in the study and were randomly divided into three intervention groups (A, B, and C), where A corresponds to TLP, B corresponds to TLM, and C corresponds to the placebo group. Strength and pain tolerance levels were measured using a handheld isometric dynamometer and an algometer. The average of three pre- and post-intervention measurements was used as the reference value for the results. Groups A and B showed improvement in pain tolerance, compared to Group C, where pain tolerance worsened. As for the gain in strength, it cannot be said that there were significant changes, the three groups showed a slight increase in strength. The presented resources are easy to apply and low cost and prove to be auxiliary tools in the treatment of patients with neck pain.

Keywords: myofascial release, trigger point, positional release, trapezius pain, shoulder

1. Introduction

Myofascial Pain Syndrome (MPS) is characterized by sensory, motor, and autonomic symptoms caused by myofascial trigger points (TPs). The myofascial trigger point is understood by a focal hyperirritability in the muscle that can strongly modulate the functions of the central nervous system [1, 2]. This trigger point can be identified by a palpable, hypersensitive nodule in a taut band of muscle. The site hurts when compressed and can produce characteristics, such as referred pain and sensitivity, motor dysfunctions, and autonomic phenomena, as TPs end up acting as persistent sources of nociceptive stimuli and contribute to peripheral and central

IntechOpen

sensitization [3]. The definition of pain was revised by the International Association for the Study of Pain (IASP) in 2020 and defines pain as "an unpleasant sensory and emotional experience associated, or similar to that associated, with actual or potential tissue damage". Being a personal experience that can be influenced by biological, psychological, and social factors [4]. Referred pain, also known as secondary hyperalgesia, is when the pain site is different from the site of its cause, it is quite common and can be found in almost all myofascial pain problems. Referred muscle pain is generally described as deep, tingling, diffuse, compressing, or pressing, differentiating it from cutaneous neuropathic pain [5, 6]. Trigger points can be classified as active or latent. PGs are considered active when they are painful with or without movement, while latent PGs are only painful on palpation. Active PGs have larger areas of referred pain than latent trigger points [7].

It is observed in clinical practice that the trapezius is probably the muscle most affected by TPs, its upper fibers produce referred pain unilaterally in the cranial direction, reaching the temporal and orbital regions, mimicking a tension-type headache (TTH). Myofascial pain in the upper trapezius region can occur due to overload and excessive use of muscles, dysfunctions, and visceral imbalances, decreased nervous influx caused by compression of the intervertebral disc and spinal roots, with or without associated physical, emotional, and dietary factors [8–10].

Positional release therapy (PRT) has as its main feature the specific positioning of body segments in order to relieve pain in sensitive points, the objective of using the technique is to benefit the patient by relieving pain and muscle spasms [11, 12]. This technique works by restoring the balance of muscle tone; normalizing fascia tension resulting in tissue relaxation, decreasing joint hypomobility as a result of relaxation of affected muscles and fascial tissues; there is an improvement in circulation and reduction of edema; pain reduction, in response to the relief of muscle hyperactivity and strength is increased because the technique can restore the tone and normal function of the muscles involved [13–15]. It is a simple, low-cost, easy-to-learn technique that is well-accepted by patients. TLP has several benefits, and in recent years it has been widely discussed and used, but it still lacks scientific studies [16, 17].

Myofascial release therapy (MLT) is a technique that works with manual mobilization of the fascia [18, 19]. These techniques are performed to reduce pain, increase local blood circulation, increase range of motion, and restore normal exercise volume and quality [20]. Therefore, TLM can be an auxiliary intervention to obtain the desired results to improve the patient's clinical symptoms [21, 22].

Given the situation presented, this research project was designed with the objective of comparing the level of pain and muscle strength in subjects with tension in the upper trapezius muscle fibers before and after the application of TLP and TLM, finally, comparing them with the effects generated by the placebo.

2. Methodology

This project is linked to the Catholic University of Pernambuco, to the Health and Life Sciences Center, to the PHYSIOTHERAPY course. Linked to the project registered under No. 442930-FTA-045-2019/5–7 and approved by the UNICAP Human Research Ethics Committee, under CAAE: 03095918.9.0000.5206 and opinion number: 140918/2018. This is an experimental cross-sectional study of a quantitative nature.

2.1 Inclusion and exclusion criteria

Inclusion criteria: (1) individuals who are between 18 and 30 years old. (2) Individuals who have neck or trapezius pain. (3) Regardless of sex, education, and socioeconomic level. (4) Who have not had a history of previous muscle injury. (5) Who have accepted to sign the Free and Informed Consent Form (FICT).

Exclusion criteria: (1) Individuals who performed strength training (bodybuilding) in the last 3 days. (2) Individuals who have a history of anemia. (3) Patients with progressive neuromuscular diseases. (4) Subjects who will undergo a previous surgical procedure. (5) Subjects who did not find PGs in the upper fibers of the trapezius bilaterally.

2.2 Intervention description

The estimated sample size was 30 subjects, who would be divided into the three intervention groups, but only eight subjects participated in the research. The eight volunteers were divided into three groups in order of evaluation. Groups A and B were composed of three individuals in each group, and Group C contained two individuals. In Group A, the volunteers underwent myofascial release therapy (MLT); In Group B, the volunteers were submitted to positional release therapy (TLP) with the positional muscle inhibition method, and Group C corresponded to the placebo group, which was performed with the application of the positional release technique (TLP) on the contralateral biceps muscle to the trapezius that was evaluated and found the main trigger point.

In the first stage of collection, an individual evaluation questionnaire was applied, which contains name, age, weight, height, gender, marital status, profession, and presence of neck pain in recent months (yes/no if yes: hours; one day ago; one week ago; 1 month ago; > 1 month. The technique to be used (Group A, Group B, or Group C). Targeting of each volunteer for the group was randomly chosen in order of volunteer evaluation: Volunteer 1 was directed to Group A; Volunteer 2 was directed to Group B; Volunteer 3 was directed to Group C; Volunteer 4 was directed to Group A; and so on, with no interference in the order in which they were evaluated.

In the second stage, the participants of the three groups underwent an assessment of the strength of the upper fibers of the trapezius using a manual isometric dynamometer (MedEOR – medtech). Subsequently, the volunteer's resistance to pain was evaluated with the Algometer (MedEOR – medtech), with pressure being applied specifically to the painful point (PG). Three measurements were performed, in which the average between them was used as a reference value (**Figures 1** and **2**).

Initially, the three strength measurements were performed, with the volunteer sitting in a chair without arms, upper limbs freely positioned on the side of the body, the strap from the equipment itself was used, which must be attached to the seat of the chair, on the ipsilateral shoulder on the side that was identified the trigger point. The volunteer was asked to shrug the shoulder toward the ear on the same side, the equipment must resist the movement. Measurements are taken before and after performing the myofascial techniques, thus recording the three initial measurements, three post-intervention measurements, and the average of the initial and post-intervention measurements as a reference for obtaining the results.

For pain assessment, the equipment is configured in its algometer mode. With the individual sitting, three measurements were taken well above the trigger point

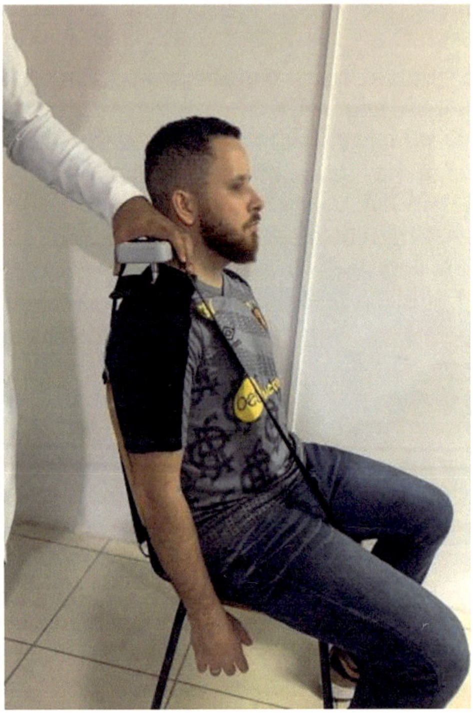

Figure 1.
Assessment with isometric manual dynamometer (MedEOR - medtech) of trapezius strength (upper fibers) with shoulder shrug movement.

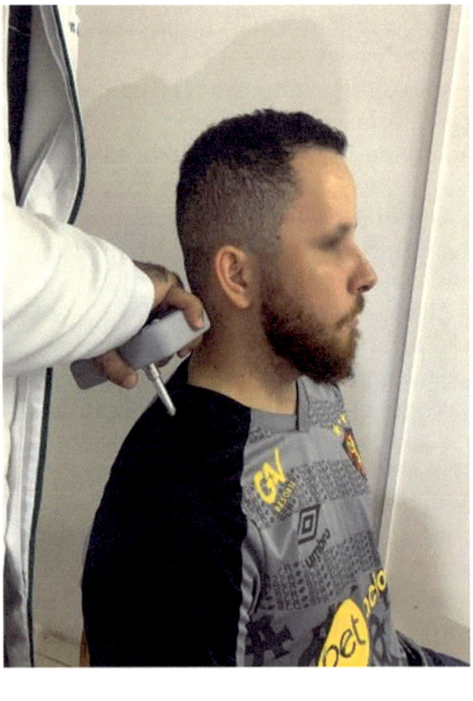

Figure 2.
Assessment of pain tolerance with digital Algometer (MedEOR - medtech) with pressure being exerted on the PG.

located, applying pressure at a perpendicular angle, until the individual reports his maximum pain threshold, thus testing his pain tolerance. Algometry showed satisfactory reliability in the results of studies on different types of musculoskeletal pain [23–25].

Then, in Groups A, B, and C, the proposed approach was performed. In Group A, superficial manual myofascial release therapy was applied. To perform the technique, the volunteer is placed in dorsal decubitus and the therapist in a cranial position in relation to the volunteer. The therapist places one finger at the occipital origin of the upper fibers of the trapezius and the other at the insertion near the acromion. The therapist should maintain the position until PG inhibition. The technique was applied until its clinical objectives were achieved (**Figure 3**) [20–23].

In Group B, TLP was applied by positional inhibition. To perform the technique, the volunteer is positioned in dorsal decubitus, with the therapist in the cranial position. After identifying the trigger point, it should be monitored, maintaining pressure on the PG, and then the volunteer's neck was passively placed in a position of inhibition, approaching the origin of the insertion of the upper trapezius muscle, passively performing an ipsilateral inclination, contralateral rotation, and neck extension. The pressure and positioning will be maintained for 90 seconds and after that time the volunteer's head must be passively repositioned in a neutral position. The theory

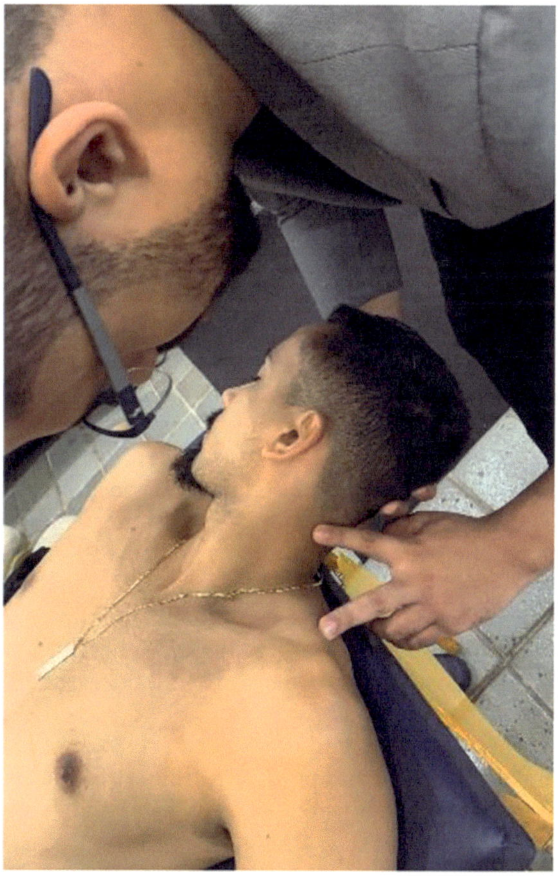

Figure 3.
Application position superficial of myofascial release therapy that was applied in group a.

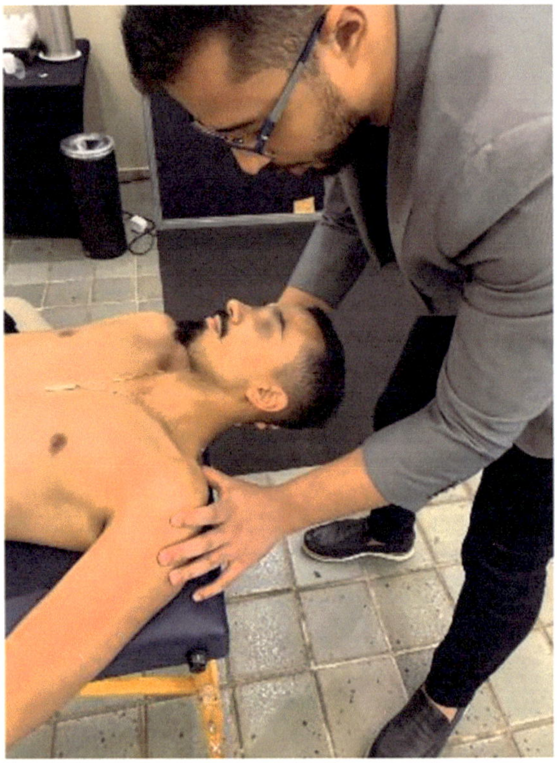

Figure 4.
Application position of positional myofascial release therapy that was applied in group B. localize the trigger point.

is that the muscle will go into active insufficiency, due to the approximation of the sarcomeres and having as a reaction the relaxation of the tissues in the region involved (**Figures 4** and 5) [12, 17].

In Group C, the control group, a TLP is performed on the biceps brachii muscle contralateral to the trapezius, where the PG was identified, in order to analyze whether the results of the previous groups are superior to the control group. To perform the technique, the volunteer is placed in dorsal decubitus, PGs must be identified in the biceps brachii muscle (contralateral to the PG identified in the trapezius) and perform their action passively, doing elbow flexion, shoulder flexion, and supination (**Figures 6–8**).

Finally, pain and muscle strength are tested again in the three groups, with the aim of comparing the results obtained before and after applying the myofascial release and positional release techniques. With this, verify if these results are superior to the control group.

Continuous variables were presented as mean and standard deviation (descriptive statistics techniques). To test the assumption of normality of the variables involved in the study, the Kolmogorov–Smirnov test was applied. Parametricity was verified in all study data. After confirming the parametricity, the data of the mean values of the Algometry in grams/force (g/f), and the results of the mean Peaks of Kg/force (Kg/f), of the tests before and after myofascial inhibition and positional release of the trapezius muscle of the study participants, the data were presented in a descriptive

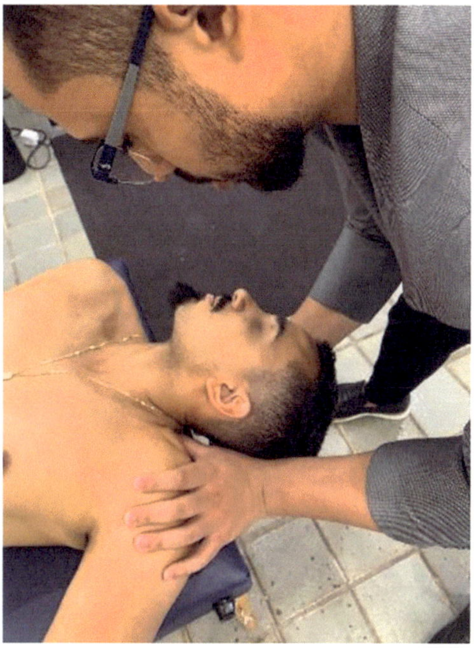

Figure 5.
Application position of positional myofascial release therapy that was applied in group B. position passively performing muscle action and hold for 90 seconds monitoring the trigger point.

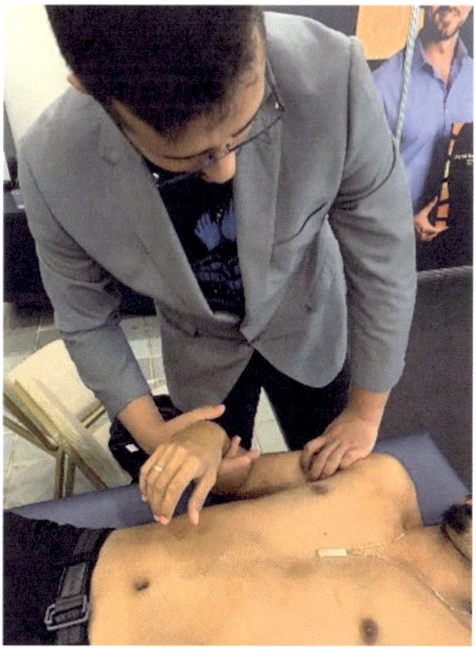

Figure 6.
Application placebo of positional myofascial release therapy that was applied in group C. localize the trigger point.

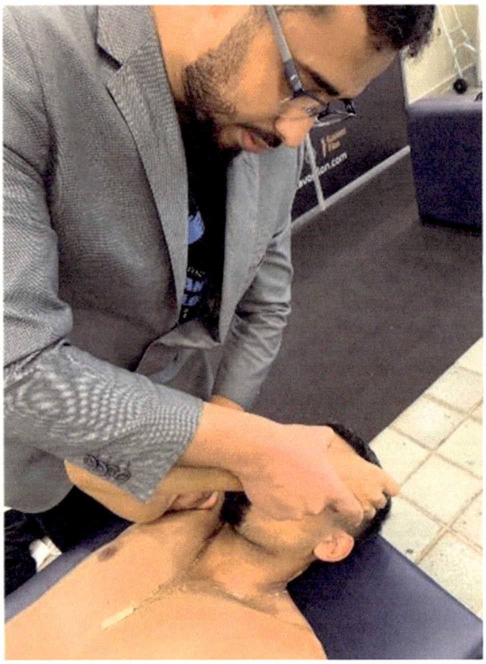

Figure 7.
Application placebo of positional myofascial release therapy that was applied in group C. position passively performing muscle action and hold for 90 seconds monitoring the trigger point.

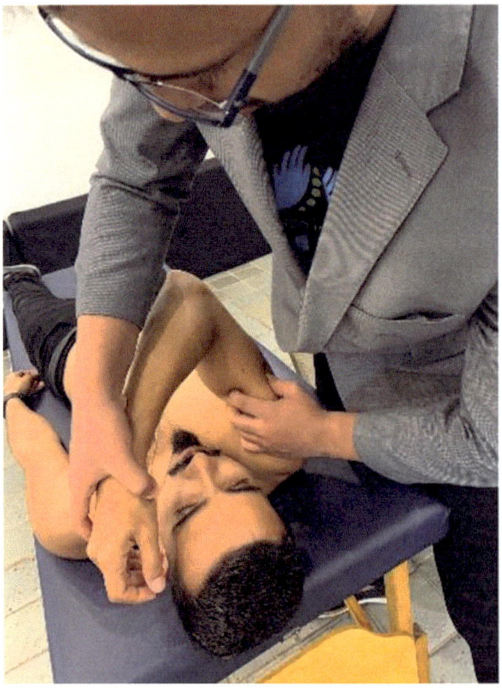

Figure 8.
Application placebo of positional myofascial release therapy that was applied in group C. position passively performing muscle action and hold for 90 seconds monitoring the trigger point.

way. The results were entered into an Excel spreadsheet and the software used to obtain the statistical calculations was the GraphPad Prism 4®.

3. Results

The sample of the present study consisted of eight individuals of both sexes, with a predominance of females, corresponding to 62.5% (i.e., 5) of the studied population.

According to the collected data, observe in **Table 1** the characterization of the public studied, the weight, age, and height data were collected in the evaluation form itself. Data referring to age faced an average of 21 years with a standard deviation of ±1.309 under the total value. The age range of the population varied between 19 and 23 years; with regard to weight, there was an average of 65.5 with a standard deviation of ±11.29, the weight variation of the individuals was between 46 and 81 kgs; the height of the volunteers ranged from 1.56 to 1.81, obtaining an average of 1.680 with a standard deviation of ±0.077, confirming the homogeneity of the group.

In **Figure 9**, it is possible to identify the comparison of the means of pre- and post-intervention results of each group related to pain tolerance (maximum threshold of supported pain), measured with a pressure algometer. According to the data collected, there was an improvement in pain tolerance comparing the pre- and post-intervention means of Group A: Myofascial Release, starting from 16575.7 g/f to 21494.6 g/f or 29.68% and of Group B: Positional Release, which presented an average of 8405.9 g/f before the intervention and 8405.9 g/f or 79.56% compared to Group C: Control Group, in which there was a decrease in pain tolerance, that is, the mean of the maximum pain threshold supported by this group was lower, since the pre-intervention mean of the group was 15,903 g/f and the post-intervention mean was 14,910 g/f or – 6.24%, demonstrating that individuals in group C endured less pain compared to Groups A and B.

	Minimum	Maximum	Average/DP
Age (Years)	19	23	21/1309
Weight (kg)	46,00	81,00	65,5/11,29
Weight (kg)	1560	1820	1680/0,077

T-test for paired samples; statistically significant difference p-value ≤. Minimum Maximum Average/DP.

Table 1.
Comparison of age, weight, and height of study participants, demonstrating the homoscedasticity of the group.

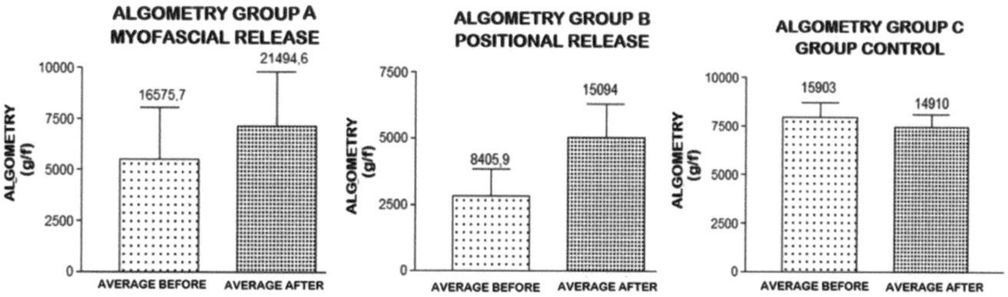

Figure 9.
Comparison of means of pain tolerance pre- and post-intervention of groups group a: Myofascial release, group B: Positional release, and group C: Control group in g/f.

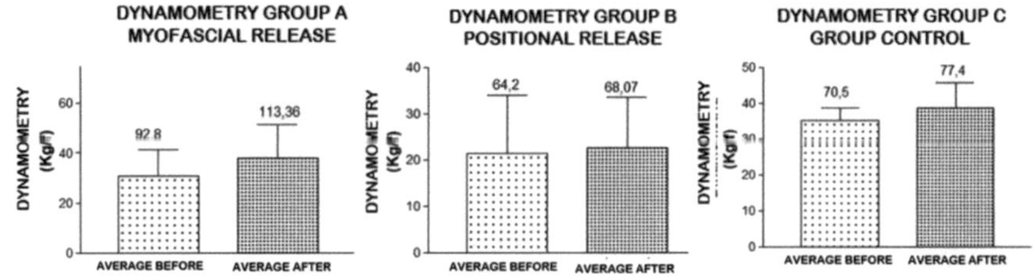

Figure 10.
Comparison of isometric strength means pre- and post-intervention of groups group a: Myofascial release, group B: Positional release, and group C: Control Group in kg/f.

Figure 10 shows the comparison of the means of the pre- and post-intervention results of each study group in relation to the strength of the trapezius muscle (upper fibers) in the movement of shrugging the shoulder, measured with a digital dynamometer. According to the data collected, there were no significant changes in Groups A and B, in relation to Group C: Control Group. However, there were gains in strength in the three groups, noting that in Group A the gain in strength was 22.16%, in Group B the gain was 6.03% and in Group C or the control group there was a gain of 9.79%, so these gains cannot be statistically significant in the present study.

4. Discussion

After low back pain, neck pain is one of the pain disorders that most affect the musculoskeletal system, when considered chronic, there is persistence of symptoms resulting in severe discomfort, absence from work, and reduced quality of life [26].

The present study was directed to investigate and compare the immediate effects of positional release therapy and superficial myofascial release therapy on the strength of the trapezius muscle (upper fibers) and on the maximum pain threshold of the same muscle. The results were satisfactory in terms of increased pain tolerance, that is, decreased pain as an immediate effect of positional release therapy (79.56%) and superficial myofascial release therapy (22.68%), but when related to strength there were no significant gains in relation to the control group.

The results of the study are physiologically justified by the study by Sain and Meena [27], it was demonstrated that positional release therapy obtains its benefits through an automatic redefinition of muscle spindles, helping to decrease muscle tone and increase the length of sarcomeres in the regions affected by trigger points. When performing the TLP technique, the muscle is positioned in its most comfortable position, resulting in tissue relaxation, improving vascular circulation, and reducing nociceptive stimuli, which are believed to be the originators of the inflammatory process. TLP also aids in peripheral and central desensitization.

Through the results, it is possible to see that they corroborate the data obtained by Namvar et al. [28], in which it was concluded that myofascial release proved to be an effective manual therapy technique in reducing pain and disability, in addition to improving isometric extension strength of the neck in patients with chronic nonspecific neck pain. In the present study, superficial myofascial release therapy (TLP) showed an increase of 22.16%, but this increase was not statistically significant because there was no significant change in relation to the control group.

In the study by Priyanka Rishi, Premlata, and Gurpreet Singh [29], it was concluded that the positional release therapy technique proved to be a favorable therapeutic instrument when the objectives to be achieved are the increase of the ROM and the improvement of the pain threshold levels in patients who suffer neck pain, in agreement with the present study.

Ravish et al. [30] compared the efficacy of the myofascial release technique with laser versus the positional release technique with laser in patients with unilateral trapezalgia. The total study sample consisted of 60 individuals divided into groups: A and B. Laser treatment was the same for both groups; Myofascial release technique was applied in Group A and Positional Release Therapy in Group B for 3 days alternately for 4 weeks. There was a significant improvement in the reduction of pain, functional limitation, and ROM., However, laser myofascial release therapy showed more satisfactory results than laser positional release therapy.

5. Conclusions

Given the situation studied, it was possible to conclude that positional release therapy and superficial myofascial release therapy were effective in increasing pain tolerance, that is, in reducing pain. However, the results did not show a significant difference in relation to strength gain when compared to the control group. The resources presented in this work are easy to apply, low cost, and prove to be tools that can help in the treatment of patients with neck pain and trapezalgia, and may precede kinesiotherapy by deconstructing kinesiophobic patterns generated by pain. Despite the numerous benefits, TLP and superficial TLM lack relevant studies and it is necessary to carry out more studies in the area, aiming at not only immediate effects but also in medium- and long-term benefits.

Acknowledgements

Thanks to the Catholic University of Pernambuco, the School of Health and Life Sciences and the university's scientific initiation, which were important parts for carrying out the work.

Conflict of interest

The authors declare no conflict of interest.

Author details

Allyson Cabral* and Paulo Veiga
Department of Physical Therapy, Catholic University of Pernambuco, Recife, PE, Brazil

*Address all correspondence to: allyson.2018109899unicap.br

References

[1] Lin T, Yeng HH, Kaziyama S, Jacobsen M. Síndrome Dolorosa Miofascial Myofascial Pain Syndrome. ATM e Dor Orofacial. 2003;**9**:27-43

[2] Batista JS, Borges AM, Wibelinger LM. Tratamento fisioterapêutico na síndrome da dor miofascial e fibromialgia. Revista Dor. 2012;**13**(2):170

[3] Travell JG. Myofascial Pain and Dysfunction/1, Upper Half of Body. Baltimore: Williams & Wilkins; 1999

[4] PAIN. International Association for the Study of Pain (IASP). Available from: https://www.iasp-pain.org/publications/pain/ [Accessed: March 27, 2022].

[5] Capó-Juan MÁ. Síndrome de dolor miofascial cervical: revisión narrativa del tratamiento fisioterápico. Anales Sis San Navarra. 2015;**38**(1):105-115

[6] Hong CZ, Simons DG. Pathophysiologic and electrophysiologic mechanisms of myofascial trigger points. Archives of physical medicine and rehabilitation. 1998;**79**(7):863-872

[7] Xu Y-M, Ge H-Y, Arendt-Nielsen L. Sustained nociceptive mechanical stimulation of latent myofascial trigger point induces central sensitization in healthy subjects. The Journal of Pain. 2010;**11**(12):1348-1355

[8] Donnelly JM, Fernández-de-las-Peñas CF, Finnegan M, Freeman JL. Dor e Disfunção Miofascial de Travell, Simons & Simons : manual de pontos-gatilho [recurso eletrônico]. 3rd ed. Porto Alegre: Artmed; 2020

[9] Calsina-Berna A, Moreno Millán N, González-Barboteo J, Solsona Díaz L, Porta SJ. Prevalencia de dolor como motivo de consulta y su influencia en el sueño: experiencia en un centro de atención primaria. Atención Primaria. 2011;**43**(11):568-575

[10] Simons DG. Review of enigmatic MTrPs as a common cause of enigmatic musculoskeletal pain and dysfunction. Journal of Electromyography and Kinesiology. 2004;**14**(1):95-107

[11] Nascimento JDS do. Avaliação eletromiográfica e clínica do uso da técnica de liberação posicional na síndrome dolorosa miofascial do trapézio. 2010. 19f. Trabalho de Conclusão de Curso (Graduação em Fisioterapia). Campina Grande: Universidade Estadual da Paraíba; 2010. Available from: http://dspace.bc.uepb.edu.br:8080/xmlui/handle/123456789/546

[12] D'Ambrogio KJ, Roth GB. Positional Release Therapy Assessment & Treatment of Musculoskeletal Dysfunction. St. Louis: Mosby; 1997

[13] de Sobral MKM, da Silva PG, Vieira RAG, de Siqueira GR. A efetividade da terapia de liberação posicional (TLP) em pacientes com cervicalgia. Fisioterapia em Movimento. 2010;23(4):513-521

[14] de Gouveia GPM. Efeito da inibição muscular na funcionalidade do trapézio fibras superiores. Fisioterapia Brasil. 2016;15(3):192-197

[15] El-Gendy M, Lasheen Y, Rezkalla W. Multimodal approach of electrotherapy versus myofascial release in patients with chronic mechanical neck pain: A randomized controlled trial. Physiotherapy Quarterly. 2019;**27**(4):6-12. DOI: 10.5114/pq.2019.87735

[16] Ritzel CH, Rodrigues PM. Terapia De Liberação Posicional e Pompage na Dor e Qualidade De Vida De Pacientes Com Cervicalgia: Revisão Da Literaturav. Anais do III Congresso Brasileiro e II Congresso Internacional da Associação Brasileira de Fisioterapia Traumato-Ortopédica – ABRAFITO. 2019;**3**(1). Available from: https://seer.uftm.edu.br/anaisuftm/index.php/abrafito/article/view/2350

[17] Mohamadi M, Rojhani-Shirazi Z, Assadsangabi R, Rahimi-Jaberi A. Can the positional release technique affect central sensitization in patients with chronic tension-type headache? A randomized clinical trial. Archives of Physical Medicine and Rehabilitation. 2020;**101**(10):1696-1703

[18] Schleip R. Fascial plasticity – A new neurobiological explanation part 2. Journal of Bodywork and Movement Therapies. 2003;**7**(2):104-116

[19] Schleip R, Klingler W, Lehmann-Horn F. Active fascial contractility: Fascia may be able to contract in a smooth muscle-like manner and thereby influence musculoskeletal dynamics. Medical Hypotheses. 2005;**65**(2):273-277

[20] Hammer WI. Exame funcional dos tecidos moles e tratamento por métodos manuais: novas perspectivas/. 2nd ed. Rio de Janeiro: Guanabara Koogan; 2003

[21] Martinez L, Plessac B. Revue de traitements des trigger points myofasciaux cervico-scapulaires. Kinésithérapie, la Revue. 2013;**13**(142):17-24

[22] de Paiva MB, Brancaleon BB, Aka JSY, Okubo ER. Modalidades Terapêuticas Alteram Limiar de Dor à Pressão de Indivíduos com Pontos-Gatilho Miofasciais. Journal of Health Sciences. 2017;**18**(4):264-268

[23] Pelfort X, Torres-Claramunt R, Sánchez-Soler JF, Hinarejos P, Leal-Blanquet J, Valverde D, et al. Pressure algometry is a useful tool to quantify pain in the medial part of the knee: An intra- and inter-reliability study in healthy subjects. Orthopaedics & Traumatology: Surgery & Research. 2015;**101**(5):559-563

[24] Montenegro MLLS, Braz CA, Mateus-Vasconcelos EL, Rosa-e-Silva JC, Candido-dos-Reis FJ, Nogueira AA, et al. Pain pressure threshold algometry of the abdominal wall in healthy women. Brazilian Journal of Medical and Biological Research = Revista Brasileira De Pesquisas Medicas E Biologicas. 2012;**45**(7):578-582

[25] Hong C-Z. Algometry In evaluation of trigger points and referred pain. Journal of Musculoskeletal Pain. 1998;**6**(1):47-59

[26] Picavet HSJ, Schouten JSAG. Musculoskeletal pain in the Netherlands: Prevalences, consequences and risk groups, the DMC3-study. Pain. 2003;**102**(1):167-178. DOI: 10.1016/s0304-3959(02)00372-x

[27] Sain M, Meena ML. Occupational health and ergonomic intervention in Indian small scale industries: A review. International Journal of Recent Advances in Mechanical Engineering. 2016;**5**. DOI: 10.14810/ijmech.2016.5102

[28] Javdaneh N, Kar AL, Faraz NK. Comparison of stability training with and without positional release technique on the pain, neck range of motion in men with chronic neck pain. Military Caring Sciences. 2019;**6**(1):49-60

[29] Premlata, Rishi P, Sing G. Effect of positional release technique versus ischemic compression on pressure pain threshold, range of motion, and headache disability in Cervicogenic headache patients among college going, students: A randomized controlled trial. International Journal of Physiotherapy. 2019;**6**(4):140-148. DOI: 10.15621/ijphy/2019/v6i4/185417

[30] Ravish V, Shridhar S, Helen S. To compare the effectiveness of myofascial release technique versus positional release technique with laser in patients with unilateral Trapezitis. Journal of Evolution of Medical and Dental Sciences. 2014;**3**(9):2161-2166